The Tropical Diet

A Scientific Simple & *Sexy* Weight Loss Strategy for Health, Sport, and Life

LISA DORFMAN, MS, RD, LMHC
America's Running Nutritionist,™
Author of The Vegetarian Sports
Nutrition Guide

Illustrations by Gary Clark, www.clarkcreativeservices.com

Visit our website *www.thetropicaldiet.com.*

Library of Cataloging-in-Publication data:
Dorfman, Lisa
The Tropical Diet™: A Scientific, Simple, and Sexy Weight Loss Strategy for Health, Sport, and Life/Lisa Dorfman.

2004091973

Includes bibliographical references and index

ISBN 0-9721985-0-4

Book production management by Sandy Dolan
Illustrations: glossary ©2001-2003, Lorraine J. Karcz
Illustrations: pyramid ©2004, Gary Clark
Author photo by Marilyn Sholin
Cover design by Andrea Perrine Brower
Inside book design by Dawn Von Strolley Grove

To my husband Bob, a Tropical Miami native

My best friend in love and in life

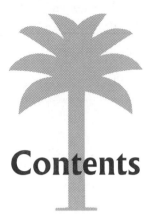

Contents

PART III: TROPICAL FOOD SCIENCE

APPENDIX

Acknowledgments

To my children, Rebecca, Danielle, and Joseph, I love you up to the clearest blue tropical sky.

To my parents, Melanie and Walter, thank you for introducing me to the tropics and allowing me to establish my home and my life here. I love you both.

To my brother Bruce and sister-in-law Dana, who live the tropical life whether sailing in the Caribbean or on Saranac Lake. Thank you for tasting all my exotic tropical foods and recipes—*Happy foods made with love!*

To my family, sister Linda, nephews Scott and Adam, niece Holly and her family, and my friends who embrace my tropical philosophy for food, fitness, and for life. Cheers.

To the Caribbean-based chefs, Chef Wolfgang Leske and Chef Lee Goble and their staff at Sandals Resorts, St. Lucia, who spent numerous hours with me to develop, calculate, refine, and prepare the delicious recipes I've adapted for this book. I am grateful for your time and expertise.

To Chef Michelle Austin, for her culinary talent and expertise and for adding spice to the book's recipes and menus.

To "Chef" Pat Vandenberg, my friend who assisted me for more than 50 hours preparing, testing and tasting recipes and for sharing some very "hot" sessions (with chili) in the kitchen!

To John Underwood, author and friend, for your generous time, your honesty and insight.

To author Jim Hall and his wife Evelyn for their faith in me, support, and friendship. To Jim for your writing inspiration, to Evelyn for your feedback, time, and expertise.

To Denise West, MPH, RD, Arlene, and all the women of the Tuesday night prayer group. To Ron and Anita Shuffield and the UBC Sunday morning study group who have prayed over my publishing efforts, my career, and family for more than a decade.

To David Kilmer, sportswriter and friend who has helped me to grow into a real writer.

And last but not least, my new friend, mentor, and editor, Erica Orloff, author, who has seasoned my writing experience with her tremendous background and expertise.

Giving Back

My first introduction to the breadth and variety of tropical foods and spices was in the early 80s. I invited a special guest to my TV show, who introduced me to a world of foods I thought only existed outside the United States.

You see, as a native New Yorker, I grew up in a meat-and-potato eating home. A glass of Tropicana orange juice was my only exposure to the Sunshine State until a trip in 1976 that changed my life. My family and I drove to Florida, and I discovered a world of palm trees, fresh fruit and vegetables, the aroma of coconut butter blending with the heat of the sun and the softness of the sand all framing the bright blue ocean water. I did not realize real people actually lived in Florida all year, aside from Mickey Mouse. It was just too beautiful a place for real-life activities. Boy, was I wrong.

Fast forward a decade to 1985.

My TV show *Food Fitness* featured guest Janelle Smith, a nutritionist with the Fruit and Spice Park located in Homestead, Florida. Established in 1944, it is the only tropical botanical garden of its kind in the United States and is residence to over 500 varieties of exotic fruits, herbs, spices, and nuts. Janelle prepared an array of exotic recipes including: tropical fruit ice cream made fresh from natural black sapote; pie from tangy, juicy key limes, and soup from fresh avocados. She also taught the audience and me about the nutritional value of these foods and published a journal article summarizing the food's health benefits. Instantly, I became excited about including these foods for patients who complained of monotony on their low-fat, low-sodium, or low-sugar diets. From there I began my research on the nutritional values of these foods and The Tropical Diet was born.

It's been almost two decades since I first introduced the program to my private patients. As a Registered Dietitian, I was able to apply the research, principles, and culinary aspects of food and balance them with the nutritional needs of my patients. Twenty years later, thousands of men and women who I have counseled for weight management, medical challenges like cholesterol reduction and diabetes, and even eating disorders, have met their dietary goals while enjoying the sensory aspects of these exotic foods, delicious beverages and spices within their normal daily diet. To date, I have used the program with recreational to professional athletes, vegetarians to carnivores, and everyone in-between.

In recent years, I had the opportunity to introduce the program to the resort industry as a spa cuisine plan. I have introduced the philosophy on cruise ships, world-class spas and resorts. As a seasoned traveler since childhood, I had an extensive understanding and appreciation for "traveling nutrition," i.e., food for leisure, eating for enjoyment. In 2000, I launched my Tropical Diet Spa Cuisine and certification program at Sandals, and other Caribbean-based resorts and restaurants so they, too, can offer healthy, fitness, or sports-minded guests healthy menu selections to control their weight, energize their vacations, and balance their typically rich vacation dining with healthy, low-fat, low-sugar, and/or vegetarian selections. The four-hour intensive workshop (for chef and kitchen staff) teaches nutrition basics, healthy cooking techniques, ingredient substitution, seasoning, safety, and sanitation issues, all geared towards giving the restaurants the power to make a difference in the public's overall health. And according to experts, the timing is right.

Chris Rollins, the Fruit and Spice Park's director since 1982, has played a key role in introducing growers, botanists, chefs, and restaurateurs from all over the world to his tropical garden of delights. Chris says, "Current interest in tropical foods is overwhelming. Ethnic fruits, vegetables, herbs, and spices can be found in local markets, gourmet shops, health food stores, and restaurants. Exotic fruits and vegetables are being mainstreamed into our menus. The Fruit and Spice Park is the only place to see and taste these tropical treats fresh from the garden."

My appreciation for Janelle's tropical nutrition lesson and Chris Rollins work for the park has inspired me to take a portion of the proceeds from this book and make a contribution the park. This donation will make it possible to provide educational resources for the public and to help to expand the park for a variety of new and exotic crops. In the end, the world will benefit from this contribution, too.

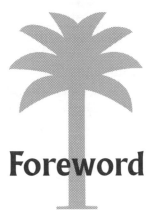

Foreword

The acceptance and availability of exotic tropical foods is a recent phenomenon in American culture. Prior to the introduction of the kiwi, the last new fruit to gain wide-scale national acceptance by the American public was the banana during the days of the clipper ships.

When I first managed the Fruit and Spice Park in 1981, tropical exotic fruits and vegetables were considered oddities. Every year the local paper would come to the Park and do a story on the quaint man growing the odd fruits. The Miami-Dade County Fruit and Spice Park exhibits more than 500 tropical fruits, spices and vegetables and has been doing so since 1944. Then, in the 1980s, things changed. Noel Vietmeyer wrote and published an article in *Reader's Digest*. He asked me if he could list the Fruit and Spice Park at the end of his article as a source for additional information. We received close to 5,000 inquiries from this story. Suddenly national publications were asking for interviews. The Fruit and Spice Park has since assisted in articles ranging from the *Wall Street Journal* and *New York Times* to *Martha Stewart Living*.

The new acceptance and interest in tropical produce that began in the 80s was due to several factors. The return of military veterans from international service, the increased ethnic presence in the United States and the emergence of affluent Yuppies, all merged into an eager market for tropical fruits and vegetables. We became more adventurous in our diet. Today this market continues to grow toward mainstream, and new produce and products regularly appear on our grocery store shelves.

Lisa Dorfman has combined exotic tropical foods and flavors with a sensible formula for health and vitality. You will learn to embrace these luscious tropical foods instead of feeling denied or restricted. Lisa's recipes utilize little-known fruits and vegetables from the tropics—as well as favorites we know and love like pineapples, bananas, and kiwi. Many of the more exotic foods, beloved in other cultures are destined to become future staples in the American cuisine.

The Tropical Diet, however, is more than adding delicious fruits and spices to your routine. It's a lifestyle. This way of eating is based upon sound nutritional guidelines. Satisfying taste and feel-good foods are mixed with a sensual program of physical and mental awareness that builds wellness. You will find that this wonderful book brings the tropics into your home. Every day can be like a mini spa vacation.

This is truly not a punishment diet. It is an opportunity to combine new and delicious food with enjoyable and sensual activities, resulting in better health and vigor. The Tropical Diet is a delicious opportunity to achieve balance and joy in your life. So if you're ready for warm ocean breezes and new foods to delight your taste buds, read on and join Lisa's many clients and fans who already know how this lifestyle can transform your world.

Chris B. Rollins
International Tropical Food Expert

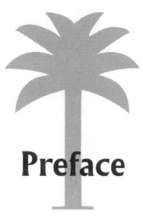

Preface

The Tropical Diet is the first weight loss program that captures the exotic image of:

A lush, warm summer breeze kissing a coconut-moisturized, tan and fit physique . . . as a radiant sun glistens off the ocean's aqua-colored waves and sparkling white sand . . . while a cool, refreshing island drink looms at the shoreline, sweating with pleasure.

There's no need to visit the tropics to appreciate the tasty lifestyle it has to offer.

Today, anyone can experience the tropics in his or her own community. Hundreds of fresh, canned, or frozen common and exotic fruits and vegetables, herbs, and spices can be found at any local grocery store. Many of the diet shakes, sport bars, and ready-to-eat meals include tropical ingredients and flavors. So you see, it doesn't matter if you live in Miami or Milwaukee, you can easily find the foods on your new program. You'll also see tropical cuisine thriving in neighborhoods and restaurants across the United States in New York, Chicago, San Francisco, and Miami. Everyday restaurants like TGI Fridays, and respected hotels such as the Four Seasons, offer tropically-dressed dishes—and why not?

Representing more than 7,000 islands spread more than 2,600 miles between Florida and Venezuela, this book presents a *kaleidoscope of colors, flavors, and tastes in fragrant and juicy recipes . . . a melting pot of Hispanic, African, Asian, Indian, and European cultures.* These foods add bold colors, textures, and flavors to ordinary recipes and lighten up the meals with healthy, low-fat tastes, garnishes, and desserts. They even help you lose weight faster. For example, kiwi, oranges, limes, and papaya consumed in precise amounts at specific times during the day can help dieters lose weight faster while maximizing the absorption of vitamins and minerals from the rest of their normal diet. These fruits and other vitamin C rich fruits and vegetables can also actually help you absorb more minerals, such as iron, from your favorite lean meats, beans, or whole grains.

While most people will think of tropical foods as fruits, such as pineapples, bananas, and citrus, this book shows readers how to create appetizing soups, salads, and desserts, which include mangos, papayas, kiwi, beans, plantains, mamey, yuca, and tomatillos. Offering a rich array of vitamins, minerals, and phytochemicals, and providing a melting pot of cultures, Tropical Dieters learn how to include these foods on a regular basis to lose weight permanently and improve their health for life. According to the World Health Organization (WHO), the U.S. Department of Agriculture (USDA), and mounds of medical research, tropical fruits, vegetables, grains, and nuts are a vital part of a disease prevention program for everyone.

How Does the Program Work?

The Tropical Diet experience can be summed up in two words: *nutritionally exotic*.

Whether you are trying to lose a few extra pounds or are training for the Olympic gold, the program shows you a plan for creating the perfect balance of tasty foods and fluids to meet your performance, health, and life goals. And on a limited calorie budget, the dieter benefits by eating more nutritiously.

And while the *science of tropical nutrition* may be complex, the translation of the science into food is simple. The Tropical Diet spells it out in three easy-to-follow programs of choice:

- The "*Lean*" low-carb, high-protein, sugar-controlled program for dieters who lose weight faster on high-protein weight loss programs.
- The "*Athlete*" high-carbohydrate, moderate-protein, low-fat plan designed for athletic training, vegetarians, or fruit and vegetable lovers.

- The "*Basic*" an even distribution of carbohydrate, fat, and protein calories for dieters just looking for a balanced nutritional plan.

The uniqueness of each of the plans is the addition of particular tropical fruits, vegetables, grains, nuts, and herbs to complement your meat-eating or vegetarian dieting preference. For competitive athletes, the vitamin C from kiwi, potatoes, and cantaloupe helps the body to absorb more of the mineral iron from meats, pork, and beans enabling them to perform faster and more intensely. Getting the extra dose of minerals from these foods can even prevent a case of anemia or osteoporosis. And those are just a few examples of The Tropical Diet's benefits.

Medical research confirms the essential health aspects of *phyto-chemicals,* "plant chemicals" also found in tropical foods. Examples are common foods you can add to your fast food meal, drink with your morning meal, and top your frozen dessert with and include onions, tomatoes, orange juice, and berries. A rich source of anti-oxidants, these phytochemicals can protect the body against "free radicals" caused by environmental and chemical pollutants and stress, which attack the cells of the system. These phytochemicals protect the body's cells and help everyone recover faster from sport training, injury, stress, and illness. Phytochemicals may also promote longevity by preventing chronic conditions and diseases.

In fact, several studies demonstrate the link between tropical foods and lower incidence of life-threatening diseases. The benefits of eating several servings of fruits, vegetables, nuts and grains each week has been shown to reduce one's risk of cancer, heart disease, and diabetes. In the long run, eating from The Tropical Diet will improve your quality of life.

Is The Tropical Diet for You?

Ask yourself these questions. Three or more "yes" answers mean The Tropical Diet may be for you.

- You've tried other popular diets for weight loss, which did not work for life.
- Now, you want a program to help you lose weight permanently and healthfully.

- You want more energy.
- You want to sleep better.
- You want a better *love life*.
- You want to live a long life.
- You have a family history of obesity, hypertension, diabetes, arthritis, cancer, or stroke.
- You've been diagnosed with a medical problem that can be easily managed with diet.
- You want to start an exercise program.
- You want to participate or excel at your favorite sport.
- You want to eat new foods that excite you, taste different, and stimulate your taste buds, digestive system, and enliven your spirits and life.

If the answer is yes, The Tropical Diet is for you. Now you can get ready for the eating experience of your life. Not only will you manage your weight, prevent or control health conditions affecting you, and learn about basic and exotic tropical nutrition, you will add a tasty spark to your life.

Just be sure to check with your physician or medical advisor before beginning any dietary, fitness, or lifestyle changes which can impact your health.

How to Use This Book

If you want to start the diet right now, turn to Chapter 4 to take your Tropical Diet Taste Test. If you want to detox first from old habits, poor food choices, sugar, fat, or alcohol go to Chapter 2. And if you want to start shopping for the delicious Tropical Diet foods suggested on the entire program, grab your grocery lists in Chapter 8. You can also log online to The Tropical Diet website to order foods directly from your home.

And, if you just want to enjoy the natural progression of the entire book, go ahead with my blessing. You've only just begun. You'll learn about the history, science, and *sex* appeal of the cuisine in the Introduction, Tropical Nutrition 101 in Chapter 4 to 6, the *L*ean, *A*thletic and *B*asic Plan overviews in Chapters 5 to 7, or if you just want to cook up some delicious food, check out the menus and recipes in Chapter 8. For those of you who are training for serious athletic events or just simply enjoy the calculations behind your program, you'll find all the equations in the tropical Energetics section in Chapter 6.

If you have any questions about the foods and the program, I've made it easy for you to get the answers. The most popular questions and answers from Tropical Dieters are included at the end of each chapter. If you don't understand a tropical "foodie" term or your questions have not been answered in the former chapters, check the Tropical Food Glossary or the appendix for additional links to tropical resources, organizations, and websites.

In the event you want a little extra personal attention and need to schedule a private appointment, you can always meet with a Tropical Diet Certified Nutritionist online privately. Just email *www.thetropicaldiet.com* with your question and a specialist will contact you to clear up your confusion.

As for now, just sit back and relax. Save your energy for the important part: the eating and exercise plan.

My personal wish is The Tropical Diet program leads you to a healthier, happier, nutritionally enlightened way of life.

Tropically Yours,
Lisa Dorfman, MS, RD, LMHC

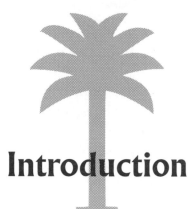

Introduction

History, Health, and Sex Appeal of Tropical Cuisine

Tropical cuisine is a rich blend of foods with a colorful history. The varieties of choices reflect the Caribbean's people, their history and politics. Above all, its dishes are always evolving, enticing, and tastefully exotic. Not only does this cuisine have a rich history, tropical foods are good for you and are endorsed by the same healthy guidelines for managing hypertension, heart disease, diabetes, circulatory disorders, and obesity. It is also a sexy cuisine filled with foods considered to be aphrodisiacs since ancient times.

The food captures the warm, white sandy beaches, ocean waves dancing with shades of aqua, green, and blue and the smell of lemon grass, frozen pina coladas, or BBQ fish all in one dish. It's like the locals—a mixture of Indian, French, Spanish, Dutch, African, and Asian descent—that all together have impacted the cuisine's evolution.

I Will Never Forget . . .

My first experience with tropical food. I was ten years old on my first cruise to the Caribbean Islands. We visited the Dutch island of Curacao; the American Virgin Island of St. Thomas, the British island of Barbados, and the Latin American coast of Venezuela. What I remember most, beyond the fresh air of the open sea and the warm breezes of the ocean air, was the celebration of food amongst the diverse European and Caribbean crew who brought fish to life with simple fruit sauces; took egg whites, and sugar to create key lime meringue into a Baked Alaskan flaming adventure; or prepared a fresh, frozen fresh pina colada dressed with a pineapple skirt to dance on the decktops with the owner of the drink. It was an adventure just to slice open my first fuzzy, fresh kiwi, and taste the bright green juicy flesh, or sample a baked calabaza pumpkin seasoned with fresh cinnamon.

Thirty years later, this multicultural experience set the stage for the profound influence of Latin, African, and Indian immigrants from Cuba, Jamaica, Puerto Rico, and 25 other islands in the West Indies and the appreciation I have for the availability of tropical foods and spices that flourish in the United States. Fifteen cruises and a multiyear contract with Caribbean resorts cemented my partnership and interest in researching the history and background of the origins of the food behind the people.

Although the basis for tropical cuisine is just steps from our shoreline, the foods, their names, and nutritional values remain a mystery to most of us. This chapter will provide a glimpse into the food's history.

Every Picture Tells Its Story

To me, tropical cuisine is *sexy*, and I'm not alone. The food screams romance, and here's why.

Since ancient times, aphrodisiac foods, substances that produced various forms of stimulation, have been shown to arouse sexual excitement in two ways: psychophysiological (visual, tactile, olfactory, and aural) and internal (stemming from food, alcoholic drinks, drugs, love potions, medical preparations). By nature, these foods represented seed or semen, or were considered inherently to have sexual powers, such as bulbs, eggs, and snails or other foods that were considered stimulating by their physical resemblance to genitalia.

The list of so-called aphrodisiacs include many foods and spices native to tropical cuisine. This earliest list included anise, basil, carrot, salvia, gladiolus root, orchid bulbs, pistachio nuts, rocket (arugula), sage, sea fennel, turnips, skink flesh (a type of lizard), and river snails. More contemporary lists include foods like bananas, asparagus, and carrots, which just happen to be shaped like sexual organs. Here are a few additional sexy foods and spices you'll find throughout the book. Many of these healthy and recommended tropical foods and beverages would make delightful companions while familiarizing you with the history and health of this delicious cuisine. Try a handful of grapes, almonds, cherries, and dates, sprinkled with a few dry roasted almonds and a bubbling glass of champagne to celebrate the commencement of your new diet program, your new way of life.

Tropical Diet List of Aphrodisiac Foods

Foods		Spices
artichokes	gingko nuts	anise
asparagus	grapes	basil
almonds	mousses	cayenne pepper
arugula	oats	cloves
avocado	okra	coriander (cilantro)
bananas	onions	ginger
carrots	oysters	jasmine
celery	peaches	mustard
champagne	pinenuts	nutmeg
cherries	pomegranates	oregano
chocolate	quince	rosemary
coffee	spinach	saffron
dates	walnuts	sage
eggplant	wine	thyme
horseradish		vanilla

Historically, tropical foods can be traced back to 4,000 B.C. when bananas, lemons, limes, oranges, and grapes were first cultivated. However, the 1400s was a turning point for introducing these foods worldwide when Christopher Columbus discovered Native American farmers growing tropical vegetables like cassava, sweet potatoes, arrowroot, pineapple, guava, and cashew fruit. And while Columbus might be responsible for introducing some of the Caribbean's staples like tomatoes, hot peppers, oranges, limes, and lemons to the Americas and Europe, Ponce de Leon played a key role by cultivating orange and lemon trees in Florida.

Probably the greatest influence on tropical cuisine came between 1518 and 1865 when more than 15 million slaves came from Africa to most of the islands. Besides bringing foods like okra, callaloo, taro (dasheen) and ackee, the Africans also developed a style of cooking which is basic to Caribbean fare. Pungent seasoning and spicing were essential to the slaves since their foods were tasteless and of poor quality. The island's English settlers added to the mix with meat, oil, vinegar, and wine and introduced these foods to the locals. Hence the melting pot had begun.

After the French and English island settlers grudgingly granted emancipation to the African slaves, they imported servants from the Orient. This group of Indians and Asians brought their traditional rice, curry, and Chinese vegetables. These foods remain an important part of Caribbean cuisine today.

Back in Europe and North America, the popularity of tropical fruits and vegetables began to grow. For a long time, only the privileged class had the opportunity to taste the delicious varieties. Advancements in refrigeration in this period also made it possible to transport foods safely back to England. This preservation method enabled all classes of Europeans to get a taste of the tropics. Now Westerners could taste the delicious flavors of bananas, coconuts, guavas, mangos, papayas, pineapples, and others once described by travelers and adventurers, who told them about the sweet fruits and their mysterious health benefits.

A few prominent business entrepreneurs took advantage of these advances by shipping fruits all over the world. Two of these businessmen later formed the United Fruit Company (UFC), one of the first fruit-growing and importing companies, and the Dole Fruit Company, synonymous with Hawaiian pineapple.

The Spices

Long before tropical fruits and vegetables were introduced to American and European cultures, tropical spices played a key role in culture, religion, and society. No other foodstuff has been at the center of so many wars and conflicts as tropical spices.

It is well known that Romans, Arabs, Ottomans, and Europeans battled with each other for control over these substances and the land and populations where they were grown. In fact, the Romans passion for spices was blamed for their collapse in 476 A.D. as their efforts to procure these special seasonings drained their precious gold reserves.

The monopolies on spices weren't broken until 1788 when a schooner from Salem, Massachusetts, secretly made its way into the Dutch Indies and brought a boatload of pepper, cassia, cinnamon, and camphor home to the United States. Tropical spices attained widespread national commercial attention into the mid-1900s with the growth of McCormick Company of Maryland and Spice Island Company based in San Francisco.

Tropical Foods in the 21st Century

Today, the United States has access to an enormous variety of tropical and subtropical foods and products. Regardless of habitat and climate, these foods are reaching all-time high numbers of consumers because of the demand from immigrants, expanding interests by culinary experts, and improved techniques and technology for processing, packaging, and transport.

Some of America's most respected chefs, including Norman Van Aiken, Alan Susser, Mark Militello, Douglas Rodriquez, and Robin Haas have popularized the cuisine in their restaurants and books (see resource section). Resorts such as Sandals, the Four Seasons, Ritz Carlton, and world-class spas regularly feature foods like mango, papaya, avocado, carambola, mamey, and key lime on their menus. Over 250 varieties of tropical foods are routinely available at most local supermarkets compared with just 50 a decade ago. And when they're not available, online companies such as Melissa's, Frieda's, Robert is Here, and others are ready to replenish your cupboards with healthy tropical dietary staples, homemade jams, and natural products from the convenience of your home. This luxury enables anyone to receive fresh mango, kiwi, guava, pineapple, papaya, okra, cassava, breadfruit, plantains, and an endless variety of fish including lobster, conch and shrimp year-round—whether you live in New Mexico or New York.

I feel privileged and fortunate to have based my home, family, and practice in Miami, one of America's largest melting pots of tropical cultures, tastes, and cuisines. It has given me the opportunity to taste and experience the foods that are the foundation for Latin and Caribbean cultures and at the heart of my Tropical Diet program.

Health Issues

Just think about it.

Wouldn't it be great if there were a diet program you can eat to:

- Lose weight.
- Train for your favorite sport.
- Feel sexy with.
- And get healthy, too.

Well, there is. The Tropical Diet will help you to lose weight and stay healthy. Just take a look at what the experts say.

The Tropical Diet's nutrition philosophy is grounded and endorsed by experts in the medical community, government, and health care organizations such as the American Dietetic Association, American Heart Association, American Diabetes Association, and the American Cancer Society. As a whole, the nutritional recommendations reflect dietary research and guidelines for preventing and managing obesity, heart disease, cancer, diabetes, and malnutrition. Many of the recommendations include healthy parameters for weight loss diets, fat intake, cholesterol, sugar, and sodium intake, alcohol, fiber, vitamins, minerals, and phytochemicals. The current dietary recommendations for managing several chronic diseases are reviewed in this chapter and are incorporated into The Tropical Diet's *L.A.B* dietary plans, recipes, and menus in Chapters 5, 6, and 7. Here's just a brief overview of how the guidelines fit into the latest dietary recommendations for obesity, hypertension, diabetes, circulatory problems, and weight management.

Obesity

Fat is a $34 billion dollar business. Powered by 97 million overweight and obese Americans, the weight loss industry is soaring. At any given time, 52 million people are on a diet.[1]

And for good reason. According to the U.S. Surgeon General, obesity has reached epidemic proportions. Results from the most recent National Health and Nutrition Examination Survey (NHANES) indicate an estimated 50 million Americans (64%) or two-thirds of U.S. adults are overweight. Among 20- to 74-year-old adults, obesity has doubled since 1980 from 15 to 31%. Five percent of America is morbidly obese.

The concerns with obesity range from the aesthetics of being fat to serious chronic diseases and even death. In fact, obesity can lead to more than 30 chronic conditions including diabetes, hypertension, heart disease, arthritis, and circulatory problems. Other conditions are listed in the Obesity-related Health Risk table.

Obesity-related Health Risks

Major Organs:

Heart
increased incidence of arrhythmias
increased blood pressure
increased resting heart rate
increased heart size
increased risk of congestive
    heart failure

Blood vessels
additional blood pathways—
    1 pound of fat
adds 200 miles of additional blood
    vessels
forty pounds adds 8,000 extra miles

vein inflammation
increased incidence of arteriosclerosis
essential hypertension

Skeletal System
Spinal column
pressure causing lower back problems
increased risk of intravertebral discs

Overall
reduced mechanical efficiency
restricted mobility
increased proneness to accidents

---

[1] Marketdata Enterprises, Inc.

Joints
orthopedic problems
increased incidence of osteoarthritis
increased incidence of gout

Muscle and Cells
reduced insulin sensitivity
impaired glucose metabolism
fat cells

Fat Cells
increased incidence of diabetes with
    upper body fat

Skin
increased incidence of ulcers, skin
    irritations, and facial hair

Brain
increase stroke incidence
risk of cerebral hemorrhage

Lungs
increased respiratory distress
sleep apnea

Stomach
increased risk of cancer

Kidneys
renal disease
hypertension

Liver
cancer
fatty liver
cirrhosis

Pancreas
cancer

Gallbladder
gallstones
cancer

Colon
constipation
cancer

Uterus and ovaries
fibroid and endometrial cancer
irregular menses
heavy menses
reduced reproductive capacity
risk with pregnancy, prolonged and
    difficult labor
increased risk of maternal and infant
    death

Other risks:
edema
susceptibility to infections
decreased sex drive
lack of assertiveness
poor self-esteem
depression
anxiety
hernia risk
operative risks
organ compression by adipose

THE GOOD AND BAD NEWS OF OBESITY

Heredity Counts

The bad news is that 66 to 80% of obese individuals inherit the condition from their parents. Poor, African-American women have the highest obesity incidence while non-Hispanic white men have a higher incidence of overweight and obesity than other groups. Women of lower socioeconomic status (SES) from all races are 50% more likely to be obese.

There is hope.

While your parents, ethnicity, and socioeconomic status (SES) may set the obesity odds against you, the good news is that dietary and activity patterns are the *primary* causes of weight gain in industrialized societies, which means you can do something about being overweight.

For instance, about 60% of Americans are inactive. According to the Department of Health and Human Services, just a minimum of 30 minutes of activity each day can make a difference in a person's weight, eating, and lifestyle habits. This modest recommendation is confirmed by other experts, too.

Another major cause for obesity in the 21st century is "passive overeating." Since so many of us live in a hectic lifestyle with joint income roles for parents, extraordinary academic demands placed on kids, and overall lifestyle time constraints, many eat out on a regular basis.

According to recent study reported in *The Journal of the American Dietetic Association,* Americans eat out 50% more than they did 20 years ago and 200% more at fast food restaurants alone. To add insult to injury, restaurant portion sizes have increased six times since 1980. Therefore, unintentional weight is gained "passively" as the consequence of time constraints, eating out, and overconsumption.

The Tropical Diet is sensitive to the 21st century's dining-out tendencies and needs. A program is in place in the Americas to educate chefs, kitchen staff, and restaurant serving staff on nutrition, healthy food preparation, and sports nutrition. Restaurants who participate in the program are eligible for the biannual Food Fitness Award in Nutrition & Culinary excellence. These restaurants will be highlighted on the *www.tropicaldiet.com* website and featured in the next book, *The Tropical Diet Spa Cuisine and Cookbook* (2005).

In the meantime, Tropical Dieters can apply any of their personal *L.A.B.* eating plans and food lists to restaurant menus since all your favorite foods are included on the program. Even fast foods are allowed on your diet! The key is portion size, condiments, and side orders. You can learn more about portion size and eating out in Chapter 8 and healthy food selection and preparation in Chapter 8.

The Tropical Diet also encourages daily exercise, whatever is easiest to incorporate and enjoyable to the dieter. Stretching, walking, even household chores will work.

THE BOTTOM LINE

To get control over your health and life and prevent or manage the chronic diseases you or a loved one deal with every day, you need to change your diet, include some daily activity, and reach your ideal body weight.

Sounds daunting. Actually your ideal body weight and healthy diet is about you. It's not about finding the best weight for your height on a chart, not about training for a marathon to get adequate exercise, or eating a specific sequence of foods.

It's about personalizing your program and goals, finding the best food, fitness, and dietary program, which helps you to become or return to your personal best for health and for life. That is what The Tropical Diet is here to help you to do. Safely, simply, and seductively so not all the fun is lost.

A DIETARY HEAD START

According to the United States Department of Health and Human Services of the National Institutes of Health (NIH), successful weight loss depends on many factors. You see, obesity is not a temporary problem that can be treated with a dietary first aid program. Weight control is about a lifelong process, one which allows you to explore your options and find the safest and most effective plan no matter what your stage is in life. The NIH suggests that any dietary program needs to include:

• Adequate vitamins, minerals, and protein.

- A nutritious low-calorie plan.
- A slow and steady weight loss, about a pound a week.

And should avoid the following pitfalls of fad diets:[2]

- Products and programs, which promise quick fixes and results.
- Any ad that says you can lose weight without paying attention to calories.
- Any plan that eschews one or more of the food groups.

In addition to these recommendations, the National Weight Control Registry[3] recorded the features of successful dieters who have lost 30 pounds or more and kept it off for at least one year. These include:

1. Combining different methods, switching around to different eating plans as long as it works and is nutritionally balanced.
   The Tropical Diet offers you three eating plans, Lean, Athlete, and Basic—all nutritionally balanced but varying in nutrient content, and the program encourages you to "switch" around when you reach a mental or physical plateau.

2. Identify a weight loss trigger. Find something that inspires you to lose weight. For men, it's often about health, aging, or sports. For women, it typically involves a love interest or emotional event such as a wedding, high school reunion, or just for "feeling" better about oneself.
   The Tropical Diet helps you to identify your most important weight loss reasons in the Detox chapter and by taking The Tropical Diet Taste Test in Chapter 4.

3. A daily exercise program, averaging 4 miles of walking each day or the equivalent.
   The Tropical Diet encourages you to exercise, any activity which you love to do on a daily basis. In fact, there are many household activities which would be equivalent to a rigorous walking program. Just check out Chapter 6.

---

[2] Tufts Diet and Nutrition Newsletter.
[3] National Weight Control Registry, University of Colorado Health Sciences Center

4. A forgiving attitude. You had a life before the diet, and you will after. Don't make your diet all or nothing.
If you can't follow The Tropical Diet daily, follow it five days a week. Take the weekends off. If you can't start a formal walking program, do something else like vacuuming the house, standing instead of sitting, stretching each morning when you wake. Don't throw in your diet towel because you can't follow the program the whole nine yards. Just think: If you exercise or cut just 200 calories worth each day, you can lose 20 pounds or more this year.

5. Monitor and measure your success. Keep track of your eating habits.
With The Tropical Diet, you can order your 30-day Tropical Diet Pocket Coach©, enough days to help you keep track of your eating, drinking and exercise for the first month. You can purchase the coaching pads through your Tropical Diet Counselor, or through the website.

So all-in-all, The Tropical Diet meets the expert's goals with flying colors. Regardless of your personal *L.A.B.* plan choice, your personal food choices from the lists, or the recipes you prepare or pick up at your local restaurant, the Tropical Diet enables you to get an adequate nutritious diet, chock-full of nutrients, protein, and fiber, which will help you shed a minimum of a pound each week while maintaining your sensuality, your social life, and your soul.

End-of-the-Chapter Questions

1. WHAT ABOUT HYPERTENSION?

Hypertension, or high blood pressure, is the third-leading cause of death in the United States. And take note of these statistics.

- Fifty million Americans over six years old have hypertension and are taking medication.
- About 28% of American adults have hypertension, a factor in nearly 70% of all cases of stroke.

- Fifty percent of those with hypertension will die of heart disease or congestive heart failure.
- Of those with hypertension, 500,000 to 1 million will have nonfatal heart related symptoms such as angina each year.
- African Americans are four times more likely to die from hypertension than other groups.

In fact, African Americans have the highest rates in the world, develop it earlier in life, sustain higher blood pressure levels, have a 1.8 times higher rate of stroke, 1.5 times higher rate of heart disease, and 4.2 times higher rate of end-stage kidney disease than whites.

The good news is that if you have high blood pressure, you can change the course of its development with a few dietary and lifestyle changes. Experts developed the following seven lifestyle recommendations and D.A.S.H. diet (Dietary Approaches to Stop Hypertension) to help those with a predisposition to hypertension or with hypertension over recent years.[4] Following the DASH diet has been shown to have the equivalent benefits of sodium-lowering drugs without the side effects or cost.

Recommendations for the Prevention and Management of Hypertension

1. If you smoke, stop smoking.
2. Lose weight if overweight.
3. Increase physical activity to 30 to 45 minutes every day.
4. Limit daily alcohol intake to no more than 24 oz. beer, 10 oz. wine or 2 oz. alcohol for men and .5 the equivalents for women.
5. Reduce sodium intake to 2,400 mg (1 tsp) day.
6. Maintain adequate intake of potassium, calcium, and magnesium from tropical fruit, vegetables, low-fat dairy and nut sources.
7. Reduce saturated fat and cholesterol from meats, fried foods, whole-milk cheeses, butter, luncheon meats, and sausage.

However, let's face it. A low sodium diet has never been sexy or

---

[4] Joint Committee on Prevention, Detection, Evaluation, and Treatment of High Blood Pressure and the National Heart Lung and Blood Institutes (NHLBI).

very tasty. Just think of the last salt-free chip or bag of popcorn you had. While The Tropical Diet incorporates all the recommendations listed, it enhances the eating experience of the hypertensive man or woman with more flavorful and colorful food choices spiced with ingredients not typically found in your hospital low-sodium cookbooks. Here are just a few of the differences you will see.

Differences between the DASH
and Tropical Diet for Hypertension

Dash Diet for Hypertension	Tropical Diet Food Servings
• 7 to 8 whole grains	tropical fruit pancakes drizzled with warm syrup
• 2 or less poultry fish or meat servings	
• 2 to 3 dairy servings	fresh fruit yogurt with granola trail mix with nuts and dried fruit
• 2 to 3 fat and oil servings	
• 4 to 5 servings nuts each week	frozen fruit sundae with a splash of orange liquor
• 5 sweets each week	
• 8 to 10 servings of fruit	berry-good smoothie with a protein blast
	raw vegetable crudités with tropical guacamole

2. HOW WILL THE TROPICAL DIET HELP MY DIABETES?

Here's an astonishing statistic: Fifteen million adults over 18 years old have diabetes. Experts say that 6 million more have it but don't know it. Who knows, this may include you or someone you love. And in 2002, the cost of treating diabetes in the United States was estimated at more than the wealth and assets of some of America's wealthiest men put together, about 132 billion dollars.

At this very moment, someone you know is taking an insulin shot or pill to control high blood sugar which leaves them weak, dizzy, thirsty, or at risk for every known chronic disease under the sun.

The problem is getting worse, not better, despite the efforts of many groups including the American Dietetic Association and the American Diabetes Association. Some of the recent advances in diet and diabetes management have shown some rays of hope. They include the following dietary interventions:

- In a recent study, people who ate whole grains were 35% less likely to develop diabetes.
- In a study of 4,898 men, even those who ate 1½ cups of whole grains a day had two-thirds the risk versus those who ate half of cup each day.
- One large Harvard study shows women who ate five palmful servings (about 1 oz.) of nuts each week reduced their risk by 27%.
- A large Harvard study of 5,103 women showed type 2 diabetics who ate fish five times week reduced their risk of heart disease by 64%, while even eating fish just a few times a month reduced the risk by 30%.

The Tropical Diet jazzes up these recommendations by showing you how to prepare delicious diabetes-safe recipes including: snapper burritos with whole grain tortillas, spa oatmeal with slivered roasted almonds and even more delicious recipes found on pages 170 to 221.

3. WHAT ABOUT MY VARICOSE VEINS?

If you're middle age, about half of your contemporaries, four times as many women than men, have varicose veins. In fact, everyone knows someone with those painful green bulging veins, tingling toes, or throbbing thighs—all examples of circulatory problems. Your risk for circulatory problems increases with age and even more so if you're obese.

And not only are they painful, they're serious. Anything that affects the body's highway of arteries and veins can even cause heart attacks, strokes, and circulatory problems such as varicose veins. I won't lie . . . diet can't completely eliminate the symptoms. However, eating certain lifestyle changes like exercise, multivitamin supplementation, and ideal body weight maintenance and eating food choices conveniently found on The Tropical Diet meets the recommendations experts advise.

These include:

- A low-fat, low-saturated fat, low–trans fat diet.
- High-fiber foods like whole grains, beans, fruits, and vegetables.

- L-arginine rich foods like fish, soy, pine, and peanuts.
- Folate-rich foods like dark leafy greens, beans, and orange juice.
- Vitamin C–rich foods like citrus, strawberries, tomatoes, and peas, which boost the production of nitrous oxide and dilate the arteries so blood flows more freely.

THE DIETARY
WARM-UP

Part I

The Tropical Diet Philosophy: The Food, Fitness, and Pleasure Pyramid©

The birth of The Tropical Diet began more than 20 years ago when I fell in love with tropical cuisine. However, it wasn't until two decades later at a spa cuisine meeting with some of the Caribbean's finest chefs that I realized what a profound influence it has had on my life. After just a few days of living the tropical lifestyle: eating fresh, local food seasoned with island spices; absorbing the aroma of lemongrass on my daily morning jogs; and drinking refreshing, iced ginger teas after rejuvenating outdoor massages, I had an epiphany. A complete state of tropical wellness was about everything the islands offered, not just the diet alone. It was at that moment I conceived the Food, Fitness, and Pleasure Pyramid©, my way of putting the nutritional aspects of this program into the perspective of an entire lifestyle.

This pyramid is my way of taking the tropical island lifestyle and packaging it in six easy steps for you to use at home. Whether you live in the Philippines or Nebraska, it will be easy for you to incorporate these steps into your lives. And when you've finished your Tropical Dieting, you've really only just begun . . . a peak nutritional experience in life.

Six-Step Program

The six steps of The Tropical Diet help you to reach your personal best: the physical, mental, and emotional place in life where food,

3

fitness, and your spirit join as one. The program adapts elements from natural medicine and applies traditional science to show anyone how to balance eating, exercise, and lifestyle to achieve harmony and peace in their personal lives.

The steps of the pyramid are:

The Earth's Natural Elements: A basis for peace, rest, and relaxation. The earth's natural elements: air and water combined with Mother Nature's sense of touch help Tropical Dieters to establish a healthy dieting balance, efficiently assimilate foods and fluids consumed daily, and reach the ultimate level of eating and living.

Food for Fuel: The nutrients found in tropical foods fuel the body, mind, and soul with clean energy for sport, health, and for life.

Invigorating Exercise: Daily activities that make you sweat. The exercise program is designed to build strength and endurance, improve circulation, memory, sleep and mood, and change your metabolism—i.e., the way the body uses and burns the calories—forever.

Tempting Tastes: A unique combination of flavors and herbs enhances the nutritional value of food and tempts your palate to experience new aromas and flavors.

Comfort Foods and Fluids: A dietary necessity . . . these are the sweet, creamy, rich and delicious treats and beverages, foods, and fluids normally forbidden on diets but necessary for lifelong weight control.

Nutritional Enlightenment: This level of The Tropical Diet is reached with the intrinsic sense of accomplishment, euphoria, and success after one to four weeks on the program.

FOOD, FITNESS AND PLEASURE PYRAMID©

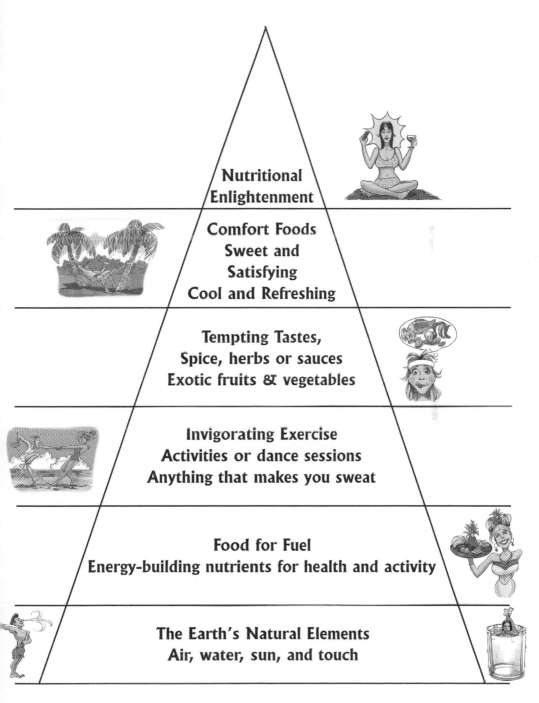

**Nutritional
Enlightenment**

**Comfort Foods
Sweet and
Satisfying
Cool and Refreshing**

**Tempting Tastes,
Spice, herbs or sauces
Exotic fruits & vegetables**

**Invigorating Exercise
Activities or dance sessions
Anything that makes you sweat**

**Food for Fuel
Energy-building nutrients for health and activity**

**The Earth's Natural Elements
Air, water, sun, and touch**

STEP ONE:

THE EARTH'S NATURAL ELEMENTS
AIR, WATER, SUN, AND TOUCH

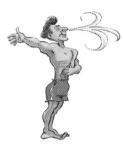

Peace, rest, and relaxation are essential for a healthy life. This portion of the pyramid emphasizes the natural aspects of your being and the earth around you. It highlights the importance of personal peace and harmony within your soul. It's simple

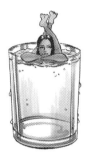

to understand and inexpensive to appreciate. All you need to do is take advantage of the earth's abundant natural resources to accomplish this goal.

Fresh air is the greatest natural gift we have. Oxygen from air assists our bodies by using the carbohydrates, proteins, and fats from food to energize our bodies, minds, and spirits. When we breathe, we can use oxygen to our advantage. We can cleanse our thoughts, recycle our energy levels, and lift ourselves from a low mental state. Breathing is essential for relaxation. Proper breathing eases tension, promotes calmness, and affects the way our bodies use and process food, as well as emotional and spiritual energy.

Think of the last time you were nervous. Your breathing was shallow and frequent. When you are stressed or nervous, your body's stress fight or flight chemicals take over to help you deal with that stressful event. Unfortunately, the shallow uptake of oxygen is just one of the ways that our system breaks down with repetitive stressful events.

That's one of the reasons why it is critical to breathe properly regardless of the day, issues, or dilemmas presented before you. It's easy to learn how to use air efficiently. Most of us just don't take the time to learn how— so let me show you.

Place your hand on belly, right on the diaphragm. Hence, this method of breathing is called diaphragm breathing. Take one deep breath slowly, and let it out at the same rate. In yoga, we count as we do this. Make sure your belly moves with each breath. Try that three times each day until you finish this book. I promise you will build your lungs and improve your endurance and energy levels. You will even learn how to cope with the distractions that can sabotage your diet, your health, and your life.

After you take several deep breaths, jog over to the kitchen and grab a big glass of water. Start right now by filling the largest mug you have with some plain water. Just think, you'll be one-eighth of the way there after you finish this cup.

Yes, water is essential for overall health, elimination, and for healing. It's the oldest form of natural therapy. Dating back to the early 19th century, Europeans built bathhouses for naturally curing aches, pains, and diseases. Walking, swimming, and bathing in water were shown to be therapeutic. Hydrotherapy continues to be a successful form of therapy today.

You need a minimum of four pints of water on The Tropical Diet— about eight cups a day. You will definitely need more fluids if you exercise, sweat, or live in a hot climate since you can lose up to two liters a day under these conditions. It only takes a 1% water loss to compromise how the body uses energy. More than 1%, and the body completely shuts down. It may even fall into an unconscious state.

Since water is the earth's most natural energy source, is inexpensive, and easy to obtain, start with water as your primary fluid first. After you master consuming water, you can graduate to sparkling waters, sparkling naturally flavored water, green tea, and organic coffee. And while the water used for hydrotherapy is very cold or hot to induce stimulation, the best temperature for consumption and assimilation is slightly cooler than room temperature.

While water does not give us calories, it does help us process, digest, and metabolize the fuel we eat, use, and expend during all activities including sleep. You can also use water to help you visualize the benefits of your nutritious foods and new eating program. Just follow along with me. Visualization therapy has been shown to treat digestive, breathing, sleep, heart, circulatory, and anxiety-related disorders and can achieve therapeutic effects, especially relaxation. Let's try it together.

Drink a big gulp of the water and swallow. Imagine it cleansing your entire digestive tract from the mouth to the colon, washing away remnants from your previous meal and the toxins of your day and past. Think of all the nutrients, the carbohydrates, proteins, and fats you have consumed through your food. Visualize the water ìdrivingî the nutrients to your muscles, liver, blood, and brain where they are processed and used to fuel your activities, thoughts, growth, and sleep. Water is a powerful natural source.

The final but not least important natural element of this level of the Pyramid is Mother Nature's sense of touch. Some see it as God's touch. Either way, touching is the basis of one of the oldest forms of remedial therapy—massage. Popular today at spas and resorts worldwide, it was referred to by Hippocrates, the father of medicine in 5th century B.C. as:

The way to health is a scented bath and an oiled massage every day.

Touching or massaging is an excellent way to relax the mind and body, which in turn enables the Tropical Dieter to use tasty food calories efficiently. It also restores balance, a sense of calmness after shock and trauma, and brings relief from everyday stresses and strains.

You don't need to get a professional massage to enjoy the comforts of touch. You can also experience touch by running barefoot on the beach, through the blades of fresh-cut grass, or the feel of cascading waters of your own shower. All of these activities provide us with a special kind of energy, a natural sense of touch to enliven our senses and spirit.

You could also be touched by your loved one, a kind gesture, or even by the warmth of the sun. Even daylight, the glow from a fireplace, or bright light can provide light and warmth, which in itself can release energy. Just think of the metabolic process called photosynthesis. This is the means by which plants trap energy from the sun to combine water and carbon dioxide to make carbohydrate energy. Sunlight can also provide mental energy, which research has shown to improve moods, and sometimes can even naturally manage some forms of depression.

If we have obtained the other elements of this step without a regular sense of touch, we risk becoming empty vessels of fuel. Touch completes the natural cycle and exchange of energy between the earth, our planet, and ourselves.

Collectively, embracing air, water, and touch can enliven your spirit, awaken your senses and prepare your body, mind, and soul for your new program and new life which lie ahead.

STEP TWO:

FOOD FOR FUEL— ENERGY-BUILDING NUTRIENTS FOR HEALTH AND ACTIVITY

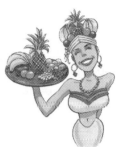

A variety of tropical foods ensures a low-fat, high-fiber daily dict rich in dense sources of vitamins, minerals, and phytochemicals. These nutrients consumed daily will help everyone to build energy, endurance, and strength while preventing malnutrition and chronic diseases.

The research that supports the connection between tropical foods and better health speaks for itself. Just look at some of the results from these large studies such as: the Women's Health Study; the British Health and Lifestyle Study; The Kuopio Ischemic Heart Disease Risk Factor Study (Finland); National Health and Nutrition Examination Survey Epidemiologic Study (NHANES); and from the Centers for Disease Control (CDC) and the World Health Organization (WHO).

The facts are:

- Those who consume fruits and vegetables three times each day compared with one time a day reduce their risk of stroke, heart disease, and death by these diseases up to 42%.
- Those who consume beans at least four times a week compared with those who ate legumes less than once a week reduced their risk of heart disease by 22%.
- Frequent consumption of berries and vegetables are associated with reduced cardiovascular disease (CVD) and longevity.
- Vegetarian women have a reduced risk of breast cancer.

• Increasing fresh vegetables and fruits decrease epithelial, digestive, and respiratory cancers.
• Diets high in fresh fruit and vegetables are associated with lower cancer rates in men and cardiovascular heart disease in women.
• Fruit and vegetable intake is inversely associated with diabetes.

In fact, in a review of more than 250 medical research reports, there was a 19 to 28% overall decrease in cancer and a 16% reduction in cardiovascular disease.

Need I say more?

The Tropical Diet's menus offer the easiest strategy for getting the most nutrient variety at every meal. You don't have to ever worry that you are getting just the right amount of protein, carbohydrates, good fats, vitamins and minerals. It's all been calculated for you. All you need to do is take the Tropical Diet Taste Test, find your personal Tropical Diet *L.A.B.* plan, pick your desirable body weight, and add a zero onto the end of that number and voila! Your perfect eating program is ready for you to begin. In fact, you can start right now!

For instance, just one cup of papaya provides just 55 calories, but has enough vitamin C to prevent deficiency and assist with eyesight. It also has enough beta-carotene to improve the sense of touch. Many of the menus are loaded with additional sources of vitamin A and C or both, and fiber, and phytochemical-rich foods such as loquats, black sapote, guavas, sapodillas. So you're never limited. Even popular fish, shellfish, lean poultry, and meat recipes provide low-fat, omega-3, protein-rich foods. To top it off, many of the foods also have a high water content, great for meeting daily fluid needs.

However, if you need more evidence, you can follow along with me here, flip over to the tropical nutrition section on pages 75 to 123, or take it one more scientific step further in the *A*thlete chapter beginning on page 85.

Either way, even if you're confident that your diet is balanced and healthy, The Tropical Diet will show you still better ways to prepare tasty, healthy foods while maximizing the meal's nutrients. To me, that is what it's all about. A key objective of the Tropical Diet is getting the biggest nutritional bang for your buck without sacrificing the taste.

Whether it means demonstrating how to select a variety of breakfast options to improve daily energy levels or how to choose innovative snacks like pineapple chunks or tropical trail mix instead of sweet pastries and chips, feel free to experiment with the food choices. Just like your favorite restaurant, the menus in Chapter 8 give you an abundance of choices for you to try out and explore different taste options. After all, if you read about the history of tropical cuisine, you know experimentation is one of the ways this cuisine was conceived. Ultimately it determines how healthy eating habits are formed.

STEP THREE:

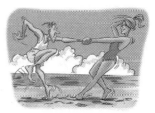

INVIGORATING EXERCISE ACTIVITIES, OR DANCE, ANYTHING WHICH MAKES YOU SWEAT

The importance of daily exercise cannot be underestimated for any weight loss, health management, or wellness program. Exercise improves flexibility, strength, and endurance; increases the body's rate of calorie use; helps everyone use more calories from fat for fuel throughout the day, and helps manage stress, stress eating, moods, and appetite. You can't lose with a little activity.

Any type of daily activity will work as long as it makes you move and sweat: from house cleaning to yoga, walking to water aerobics. The key is to get the heart rate up and sweat. Here's why.

Your heart is a muscle. So is your skin. The skin actually has two to four million sweat glands. Believe it or not, your feet actually sweat the most!

The skin is sometimes called the "third kidney." It is far more complex than the kidney or any other organ except the brain. It's composed of blood vessels, nerve endings, and vessels for carrying lymph, pigmentation, oil glands, hair follicles and cells that waterproof and deny bacteria entry to the body. And of course, it is home to the sweat glands.

Hear me loud and clear. **Don't be afraid to sweat.** On The Tropical Diet, it's actually recommended. Sweating is therapeutic, and here's why. Sweating is as essential to our health as eating and breathing. It accomplishes five important tasks:

- It rids the body of wastes (see Chapter 3).
- It regulates the body's temperature of 98.6 degrees F.
- It keeps the skin clean and pliant.
- It has a relaxing effect.
- It gives relief from the common cold, arthritis, headaches, and hangovers.

It's a fact that sedentary people don't sweat enough. That's one of the reasons why a sweaty workout each day is so important. In fact, a physically idle lifestyle, antiperspirants, artificial environments, smog, and synthetic clothing all clog skin pores and inhibit the healthy flow of sweat. These detrimental effects are reversed when you allow your body to sweat.

Sweat is also a great detoxing agent (Chapter 3) Ninety-nine percent of what sweat brings to the surface of the skin is water, but the remaining 1 % is mostly undesirable wastes. Excessive salt carried by sweat is generally believed to be beneficial for cases of mild hypertension. Urea, a metabolic by-product, also needs to be eliminated and can be accomplished by a good sweat. If not disposed of regularly, urea can cause headaches, nausea, and in extreme cases, vomiting, coma, and even death. Sweat also draws out lactic acid, which causes stiff muscles and contributes to general fatigue. Sweat flushes out toxic metals such as copper, lead, zinc, and mercury, which the body absorbs in polluted environments

Tropical Dieters who engage in regular activity will see their diets in action. They will have immediate physical and mental effects as a result of sweating and training. They will undeniably look better as they lose weight. Regardless of the dieter's level of fitness, pain threshold, or age, there is never an excuse not to exercise. Dozens of activities, classes, and sports are offered in health clubs, community centers, on video, and on TV worldwide.

STEP FOUR:

TEMPTING TASTES: SPICES, HERBS OR SAUCES, EXOTIC FRUITS OR VEGETABLES

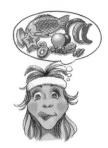

If you have ever visited the Caribbean islands you know the foods are an enticing, exotic blend of cultures and tastes. And while the United States is situated relatively close to the islands, the cuisines remain a mystery. In two words, it is *tastefully exotic.*

After working with world-renowned chefs from Germany and England in St. Lucia, Jamaica, the British Virgin Islands (BVI) and elsewhere, I have learned there are many ways to prepare the same combinations of foods and spices without getting bored. And while you may get ideas from the recipes in this book, the truth is you can make Tropical Diet dishes hundreds of ways and make them all taste good. You can never get it wrong.

The most appealing features of any meal are the tempting tastes, spices, and sauces which enhance the food's appearance, color, texture, and aroma. Once you experience Tropical Diet meals, you'll never forget it. In fact, research published in *The Journal of the American Dietetic Association* demonstrated how important the chemosensory stimulation from the food I am describing is, which can have profound influences on metabolism, nutrient-absorption, and appetite. Some even refer to this phenomenon as *Umami,* the fifth taste—tasty, meaty, savory, or just plain delicious[1]

Tropical Dieters will find this cuisine easy to prepare. The simpler the cooking process, the more nutritious the meal becomes. Just think, the beauty of most of the islands is simple cuisine without the aid of microwaves, food processors, fancy knives or utensils. And as a result the foods taste better, too! So you also do not need to buy much equipment to prepare this cuisine. In fact, a frying pan, some tinfoil, a knife, and a measuring cup will do. You see how easy it's going to be to prepare delicious meals!

---

[1] Wine Spectator, 2003.

STEP FIVE:

COMFORT FOODS: SWEET AND SATISFYING, COOL AND REFRESHING

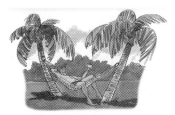

You heard it here first. It's sexy to eat and drink forbidden foods! And normal to desire them too! In fact, repeat after me,

> *It is normal to enjoy comfort foods and beverages at any stage of life.*

Sweet foods and drinks are soothing, fun, and pleasing to the tummy and mind. Sweet foods actually release a brain chemical called serotonin which has a relaxing and calming effect on the body. Alcoholic beverages, particularly cordials, daiquiris, and wine also help to relax the body. A daily glass of red wine may even reduce the incidence of heart disease in some individuals.

Take away dieters' favorite sweet and comfort foods, and at some point they will crash mentally and physically, especially those who have been following high-protein, low-carbohydrate diets for extended periods of time. Research has shown these folks especially crave sweets and suffer from rebound weight gains as a result of their skewed dieting regimen. Hence, I believe it is healthier to include a few sweets over the course of your diet than no sweets at all.

And according to the Fruit and Spice Park director, Chris Rollins, *tropical fruits are nature's best sweets.* The Tropical Diet therefore naturally builds in sweet foods to all the plans, even the *L*ean program, which is technically lower in carbohydrates than the other two programs.

A word of caution.

While sweet foods and drinks are desirable from time to time, they are not recommended on a daily basis for anyone, even athletes, and certainly not in excessive quantities. And while some individuals will continue to indulge in sweets and alcohol on occasion, it is important to balance your sugar and alcohol toxicities with plenty of water, non-alcoholic beverages, and fluids from fresh fruits and vegetables to prevent dehydration and the side effects of hangovers.

STEP SIX:

NUTRITIONAL ENLIGHTENMENT

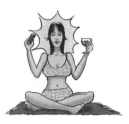

And in the end . . .

The Tropical Dieter will attain a higher state of consciousness I call nutritional enlightenment. It is a state of euphoria where your body rejoices after you follow the first five steps of this pyramid.

Psychologist Abraham Maslow referred to attaining the highest level of needs and desires in life as self-actualization. To him, this level reflects the desire to become everything we arc capable of becoming, the urge for self-fulfillment. Nutritional enlightenment is my dietary version of self-actualization. You actually become your personal best in every way.

Sometimes this euphoria is short-lived as a passing moment. It may also stay for a few hours after a morning workout. If you're really fortunate, it will reside in you forever.

This enlightenment will also spread to other areas of your life, inspiring you to succeed in relationships, work, family, and athletic performance. And while your personal goals, dreams, and desires may change as you mature, you will never forget The Tropical Diet's effect and the valuable lessons that will stay with you for the rest of your life.

The Tropical Diet Detox

The Tropical Diet detoxification plan is necessary for everyone who wants to lose weight permanently. For the average dieter, the detox phase of The Tropical Diet will only take a day or two, so don't skip it. For some it may take up to ten days to clear the toxins from your body, mind, and soul.

Either way, think of it as a means towards cleaning your personal "poisons," a.k.a. the damaging ingredients, habits, behaviors, and lifestyle patterns out of your life. Detoxing two to three times each year will rejuvenate your energy levels and help you start a new cycle of eating. Think of it as your dietary seasons of change.

A Dietary Reality Check

Detoxing is not easy. In fact, the detox will challenge your commitment and patience for the Tropical Diet. Doing the detox means that you will have to face your personal nutritional demons. And no one likes to face their worst eating and lifestyle traits.

But trust me, it will make your Tropical Diet success that much sweeter. Just think, the eating behaviors, obsessions, and compulsions to food, additives, drugs, and behaviors will be gone. You'll also get rid of some of the consequences of those habits such as headaches, joint pain, indigestion, bowel disorders, excessive lethargy, body stiffness, and

17

personal and emotional stagnation. And this is just a partial list. Additional symptoms are listed in the Detox Questionnaire on pages 24 to 26.

Several Eastern philosophy religions and medical systems advocate detoxing weekly, *naturopathy,* the umbrella term used to describe a range of natural therapy treatments and *Ajurveda,* the "science of life," believe detoxing or fasting is physical necessity for cleansing the body of poisons accumulated from poor eating, the environment, and/or suppressed or repressed emotions. They also recommend it for enhancing the immune system and speeding up the healing process, i.e., "starve-a-cold" philosophy.

Why Detox Now?

The detox will help you to graduate to better eating habits while following The Tropical Diet. Think of it this way. If you were promoted to a new position at work, would you want to keep your old office? Of course not. You would want a new office, a new environment to "house" your new position. Well, it's the same with a diet.

The detox encourages you to permanently change the house where your diet will be residing. Hence, it'll be harder to regress back to old eating habits. A benefit of the detox program may be to avoid one of the common pitfalls of dieting. Research proves that when dieters return to former eating habits, their weight and cravings are more difficult to control. The detox may help you make The Tropical Diet your last weight control program.

It's also important to detox now before you really start to show signs of aging. Here's why. While it was easier to eliminate alcohol, sugar, and other substances while you're young, the body gets less efficient at "clearing" the toxins as we age. How difficult is it to stay up late or to have a few drinks compared to your younger days? Admit it. Each year, you get a little more sluggish as you try and push the limits of your stamina for a special occasion.

With too many late nights, alcohol or food binges, your body suffers unnecessarily from the additional stress. Consequences include the short-term effects of the awful morning look—puffy eyes, headaches, and lethargy—to long-term effects such as clogged digestive tracts and arteries.

These effects are not a surprise since the stress–diet link is one of the leading causes of "clogged" physical ailments such as constipation and hypertension. If left unaddressed, these conditions can develop into more serious diseases like colon cancer and heart disease.

Behavioral research shows excessive work, exercise, and emotional trauma can also cause toxin buildup. The body has to work extra hard to keep up in these situations and defends itself with metabolic side effects to keep the body homeostatic or balanced. The body then expels these toxins through the lymphatic system and blood, skin, bowels, lungs, kidneys, and liver. However if this sort of indulgence is a repeated pattern, the body fails to keep up. As a result, you suffer with the emotional toxins of lethargy, grogginess, emotional heartache, depression, and chronic fatigue.

While most people can benefit from detoxing, there are others who should not practice this regimen. Poor candidates include pregnant or breastfeeding women, children and teens, individuals with emotional or eating disorders, or those on prescribed medications.

What Are the Primary Goals with the Detox Phase?

The primary goals of this phase of the program are to ensure your long-term success on The Tropical Diet. Some of the major reasons for detoxing include:

A HABIT CLEANSE

To break food obsessions, habits and cravings and food jags . . . both *healthy and unhealthy foods* consumed compulsively and on a regular basis.

If the foods compulsively eaten contain excess fat, sugars, and calories, they're likely to cause excess weight, body fat, and numerous medical conditions. If the foods are enhanced with sodium, or preservatives, even fiber, you might experience a number of other consequences such as puffy eyes, swollen hands and feet, insomnia, nervousness, skin conditions, and a depletion of the body's vitamins and minerals.

Here's a good example of a habit cleanse I needed to endure during college. In order to get through graduate school, we needed to go through the process of dietary modification ourselves so we could learn to relate to the clients we would soon counsel. I was a fairly good eater, however because of my hectic school schedule and marital responsibilities, I had a bad habit of skipping breakfast and lunch and eating most of my calories during the evening. Maybe you can relate.

In fact, for most of my life, I skipped breakfast and lunch in lieu of work and chores so I knew this lifelong habit would be the most difficult change I would ever make in my life. Even harder than adjusting to marital life at 21 years old! I knew it was something I needed to do, especially if I was going to counsel others to do the same. Where was I going to begin, with the afternoon or the morning meal?

Here's what I did.

Since actually eating a sit-down morning meal was going to be nearly impossible, I decided to pick up some shakes at the store. I figured out that 250 calories of a nutritious beverage was equally as good as chewing away at toast or eggs. I also tried joining my husband at the breakfast table with his morning cup of coffee. I didn't drink coffee, however, I made myself a café con leche, a Latin-style brew with mostly milk. The cup of milk in the coffee would serve as a breakfast-item alternative to the shake. Remember it was the routine and habit of having some form of calories in the morning that was important.

Then I did the same for lunch. Liquid calories. I stopped for a smoothie, frozen yogurt, or sports shake, which eventually graduated into the drink with a side of fresh fruit or crackers. So you may wonder what impact this had on my evening meal.

A huge impact.

I wasn't as famished at night after work. My calories became more evenly distributed, my meals better planned. The bad habits I detoxed out of my life and the good ones I incorporated into my daily activities prepared me for three healthy pregnancies and a twenty-year career in competitive running, triathlons, and multisport events. I have never looked back and continue to have a minimum of three meals a day and feel great.

Assist with Withdrawal

. . . from caffeine beverages, alcohol, diet foods and drinks, over-the-counter medicines and diet pills and recreational drugs. While this group is more challenging than other groups because they involve neurotransmitters, nerve chemicals in the brain that grow accustomed to having these chemicals stimulate emotions, actions, and feelings, it is not impossible to naturally detox from them, and it is a vital part of your success.

Environmental Pollutants

. . . food toxins from herbicides, hormones, pesticides, viral, bacterial contaminants which infect the food supply. These can include every aspect of the food production process including the animal feed, watering system, transportation, handling, and shelf life. Environmental pollutants may cause allergies, headaches, mood swings, cramping, dizziness, and bowel problems, and they constitute a hidden contaminant often unseen and unappreciated by the public. While it is not essential to give up the products in this group (and often impossible), for those on the healthier end of the spectrum with little to detox from other groups, eliminating some of the foods and beverages from this group may enhance energy levels and overall health in the long run. All you need to do is replace some of your everyday snacks, cereals, and beverages with organic, natural, or free-range ingredients or animal products.

Supplements

Vitamin and mineral supplements, bars, and shakes can also become addictive requiring the body to become accustomed to a higher intake for health maintenance. A good example is vitamin C. More than 100% of the RDA for this vitamin may be toxic for some individuals. Detoxing off this supplement will help you adjust to a more realistic lower requirement rather than the supplement dosage amount. This will help anyone consuming too much vitamin C and other vitamins and minerals save money and the dependence to excessive amounts.

MEDICATIONS

Over-the-counter medicines, pain relievers, cold remedies, and allergies/sinus medications can also become addicting, unnecessary, and cause undue side effects such as rebound headaches, higher dosages required for effectiveness, and a pure addiction to the substance to maintain daily living functions. Advil and other medications can cause liver damage, stomach problems, and bleeding ulcers, all serious and life-threatening side effects of these seemingly innocent drugs. All of these can be detoxed from the body to avoid dependence and to stimulate their action when needed for legitimate reasons. This is of course barring any health problems or recommendation by your personal physician.

EMOTIONAL CLEANSE

Sometimes we need a time-out, even as grown-ups. The daily stress of life, environmental noise, work, and family responsibilities stress our mental capabilities, our physical stamina, and spiritual peace. If you're fortunate enough to have the time, money, and freedom to take an extended vacation, go for it.

Whether you're financially able or not, finding ways to get away from it all is a must for keeping a healthy balance and perspective on life. Some ways you can take mini-breaks from the grind of work, house chores, and carpools, or even the responsibilities to church, community, and school is by setting aside a few minutes each day to be alone with nature, with your god, and with yourself. Practice your deep breathing exercises described in Chapter 1. Take a walk or jog at sunrise. Meditate at sunset. Read your devotional book, prayer guide, or favorite novel by the fireplace.

I take many detox time-outs during the week. Since my time is limited by being a wife, mother to three teenage children, and a full-time career woman with an active website, there are few places I can hide during the average day.

Some things that help me take a break are:

• Waking up at the crack of dawn before the world has the chance to catch up. Sometimes I meet friends to run, swim, or cycle or sometimes I go alone. This peace first thing each day helps me collect my thoughts and face the tasks I have ahead.

- Working on jigsaw puzzles. I find this activity relaxing and challenging all wrapped up in one. I will keep a puzzle on an unused table in my home and take a five-minute or one-hour break each day to focus on that puzzle and nothing else. This helps me clear my thoughts and renew my energy for chores and responsibilities waiting for me to attack. If I find a piece or finish the puzzle, I really feel a sense of accomplishment.
- Reading the Bible and perhaps even attending a Bible study. Regardless of your religious background, studying about your spiritual background with others often gives me a sense of purpose and direction with people who have the same beliefs. And just when I think I have too much pressure or stress in my life, I read about some of the Bible characters who literally had the world on their shoulders and I feel my issues are small in comparison. Studying the bible with other women at Bible Study Fellowship (BSF) or in private homes gives me the rare opportunity to connect with other women willing to share and confess the issues we deal with as mothers, wives, and professionals. I find that many of the challenges we all face get resolved with a faith-driven outcome.

How Do You Know If You Need a Detox?

Some questions you can ask yourself.

The following questionnaire will give you an additional resource to assess your need for detoxing. The higher your score, the greater your need.

	Never	Sometimes	Often
1. You feel lethargic, tired, and drained on a daily basis.	0	1	2
2. You feel less than your best despite the decency of your diet, exercise regimen, and supplement regimen.	0	1	2
3. You wake up stiff in the morning.	0	1	2
4. You wake up with puffy eyes, hands, or legs, or experience fluctuations in your extremities and eyes during the day.	0	1	2
5. Your mood is worse more of the time than better, regardless of your work schedule, stress level, home or family responsibilities.	0	1	2
6. You have difficulty sleeping at night and staying awake during the day.	0	1	2
7. You have stomachaches, indigestion, or nausea after eating regardless of your food choices.	0	1	2
8. You have hard, difficult, or infrequent bowel movements, or too soft, foul-smelling excessive bowel movements.	0	1	2

	Never	Sometimes	Often
9. You catch colds, more than one to two episodes each year.	0	1	2
10. You have allergy symptoms like congestion and headaches or sinus problems.	0	1	2
11. You get injured frequently or do not recover well from everyday chores.	0	1	2
12. You are depressed and have a difficult time looking forward to each day.	0	1	2
13. You have a strange body odor other than perspiration.	0	1	2
14. Your urine is dark, not nearly clear, smells, or is difficult or painful to pass.	0	1	2
15. You have bad breath, a bad taste in your mouth, or burp frequently.	0	1	2
16. You pass gas frequently, more than a few times each day, and not due to the intake of high-fiber foods.	0	1	2
17. You have difficulty concentrating, remembering easy facts, or focusing.	0	1	2
18. You have brittle nails, your hair falls out, or your skin and eyes are dull, red, and blotchy or greasy.	0	1	2

	Never	Sometimes	Often
19. You are anxious over minor issues or over issues that are not in your personal control.	0	1	2
20. You have swollen lymph in your neck, under your arms, in your groin.	0	1	2
21. You suffer with daily or frequent headaches.	0	1	2

RESULTS

If your score was higher than a ten, it means you need to follow the detox plan for a minimum of a day before commencing on your Tropical Diet Personal Plan.

A score greater than fifteen may indicate a more serious health problem. Therefore, if you have not had a full medical checkup including the following tests, call your doctor right now before starting this or any other diet program:

- Blood examination.
- Complete blood test and CBC.
- Pap smear.
- Colonoscopy (over 50, or younger with a family history).

Speak to your physician about your dietary plans. Receive a letter of approval before beginning The Tropical Diet or any diet program.

GETTING STARTED

In order to plan a healthy detox, here are a few tips to get the ball rolling. First of all, you'll need to do the following:

1. Choose the date to begin.
2. Prepare loved ones by sharing your detox schedule and your expectations from them, e.g., no entertaining, social

engagements, or unnecessary road trips. Choose a time that is ideal for your family to ensure better success.

3. Purchase the foods, fluids, and supplements from the lists on pages 133-141.

4. Clear your mind of work projects, deadlines, and commitments.

5. Plan for withdrawal. Some of the symptoms you may experience could include: headaches, lethargy, and a bad taste in the mouth. You may also be cranky, easy to anger, or excessively energetic. Both may compromise your work and family life.

6. Be prepared to go to the bathroom frequently. No cross-country car vacations or marathon training during this time. Expect to drink 3 to 4 pints of fluid each day.

7. Buy extra air fresheners and bathroom spray. Your bowel movements may smell more foul than usual. The liver's conversion of waste materials may account for the funny odor. Some may include a smell of ammonia from excess protein waste, recreational and over-the-counter medications, alcohol, inhaled toxins, and foodborne toxins.

8. Do not go headstrong into the detox. You may benefit if you eliminate each of your personal toxins over a 3 to 10 day period, particularly if you've been adhering to them for months or years. You may even want to work on one habit, start your Tropical Diet *L.A.B.* plan, and then resume a detox for another habit. No need to build Rome in a day!

DETOX STEPS

- **Detox Step One.** Eliminate your priority physical or mental intoxicant, e.g. alcohol, sugar-laden, fatty, fried, or fast foods. Do this for the first 24 to 48 hours. If you feel better, proceed. If you feel side effects to your withdrawal, continue with this same elimination for another 24 hours. When you feel better, you can take Step Two.

- **Detox Step Two:** Eliminate your secondary toxin, e.g. dairy, wheat gluten, processed foods, recreational drugs, over-the-counter medications, supplements, and lifestyle habits. Eliminate this habit for the next 24 to 48 hours until you pass the toxin and no longer suffer from crankiness, headaches, lethargy, or anything else abnormal. Afterwards, you may proceed to Step Three.

- **Detox Step Three.** Begin including 3 to 4 pints of fluids, sparkling water, green tea, or herbal teas. Make sure the teas are nondiuretic, i.e., do not contain senna, cascara sagrada, aloe, rhubarb root, or buckthorn, since they can cause serious diarrhea. Choose any of the fresh, diluted Tropical Diet Detox cocktails (page 32) or mix ½ cup of your favorite organic juice with ½ cup sparkling water. Drink these three times each day, ½ hour before mealtime.

- **Detox Step Four.** Follow the specific Detox Diet listed on page 33. Include one to two detox food servings from each food and herb category on page 34.

- **Detox Step Five.** Grow or purchase fresh herbs such as peppermint, ginger, or oregano. Include them in your daily detox recipes.

If you choose to stay on the detox for more than one week, include a minimum of 1 cup of brown or wild rice, quinoa, legume, rice or potato-based pastas, plain potatoes, couscous, millet, or polenta two times a day in the afternoon and early evening.

Phase One
The Tropical Diet—Detox Eating Plan

PREPARING FOR YOUR DETOX:

First, write down your top three dietary pitfalls and behaviors. It may be obvious which habits hold you back from being your personal best. Other habits may not be so clear to you.

Refer to Table 1 for help with this.

1. _____

2. _____

3. _____

Some of the most common toxins and habits can be found in Table 1 below. Remember, a food or habit can initially be a healthy addition to your life then become a toxic ingredient if you overindulge in that behavior. So, don't be surprised if you see foods like yogurt or wheat bread.

Table 1
List of Common Toxic Foods, Behaviors, and Habits

Candy
Ice cream
Cordials
Sport bars and drinks
Sport gels
Chewing gum and hard candies
Chocolate

High-fat foods
Fried anything, even vegetables
 and fish
Fast food
Sandwich meats
Butter, lard, and oils
Desserts
Bacon and sausage
Sandwich meats
Frozen food meals
Cheese
Dairy—whole milk, whole yogurt,
 and cream
Chocolate
Chips
Nuts

High-carbohydrate foods
White or whole-wheat bread or rolls
Muffins, doughnuts, cake, cookies
Pasta
Potatoes
Rice
Crackers

Chips
Popcorn
Pretzels
High-sugar foods
Cake

Toxic substances
Alcoholic beverages
Diet sodas
Recreational drugs
Over-the-counter drugs and medicines
Prescribed medicines when no longer
 needed, i.e., pain pills,
 anti-anxiety pills, or antidepressants
Diet pills, or ephedrine, guarana, and
 other natural diet pills

**Chemical additives and
 preservatives found in**
Cereals
Crackers
Snack foods
Baked goods
Chips
Pretzels
Dairy
Juices
Sodas—diet and regular
Frozen meals and foods
Candies

And seemingly healthy food choices and habits

Vitamin and mineral supplements

High-fiber foods and supplements

Air-blown popcorn

Diet shake and bar addictions

The need to eat the exact foods and meals every day

Sugarless chewing gum and candy

Dietetic candies, frozen meals, and treats

Intense exercise sessions

NEXT . . .

The next step is to eliminate those foods and habits from your life. Take a personal action plan and stick to that plan even if the withdrawal symptoms seem impossible to overcome. You can get additional support and assistance from family, friends, neighbors, clergy, support groups, and even from the *www.thetropicaldiet.com* website.

For example if you:

Food Choice or Habit	Consequence	Plan of action	Accomplished (✔)
Have a daily alcoholic drink	weight gain	stop drinking today	in 3-days
No vegetables or fruits in diet	constipation	include 1 serving fruits/vegetables/ day from Detox list each day	in 3 days
No exercise	unfit/excess body fat	Start a walking program today	1 week—walking 30 minutes each day
Eat one meal/day after 6 pm	poor sleep; excess body excess caffeine intake during day for energy	include one healthy food or beverage from the food list i.e. apple, at 1-2 times during each day—morning & afternoon;	1 week including snacks and reducing meal size
Large evening meal	poor sleep; weight gain	Reduce meal size at evening meal by reducing portion sizes of protein or starch, i.e. ½ chicken breast instead of whole; 1 baked potato instead of French fries and dinner rolls	1 week of monitoring portion size, and monitoring eating habits

FINALLY . . .

Reward yourself. Rewards come in all shapes and sizes so it doesn't need to be expensive. In fact, *intrinsic* rewards include the inner accomplishment such as just feeling good about your new lifestyle. To reinforce your success, you can hang a positive poster on your refrigerator or journal your new habits.

Rewards can also be *extrinsic*. These rewards include the new outfit, present, or trip to the spa.

Your best reward will be the present of health you give to yourself. By detoxing your obsessions, compulsions and ugly habits, you escape from your personal prison, the chains which have been holding you back from being your personal best.

Congratulations to the new you!

DETOX FOOD CHOICES AND MENU

The detox food lists and menus are intended to:

• Cleanse and detox the gastrointestinal tract.
• Encourage fluid elimination.
• Inspire perspiration.

You need to follow the menus as closely as possible. If you feel any side effects that concern you, call your physician or emergency personnel immediately. Remember, you are the best judge of your body, therefore you need to be in charge of its best health and care.

Detox Daily Guide

WEEK ONE

During the first week of the detox, you need to consume a detox tonic each morning to assist you with a wake-up cleanse. Try all of the detox tonics until you find the best and tastiest one for you. To this tonic, add one tablespoon of ground flaxseed to get a good source of omega-3s.

Wait a minimum of ½ hour after drinking your tonic before consuming your morning meal.

Your choices for the morning tonic are:

• A cocktail of warm juice and lemon.
• One cup bottled water mixed with one cup organic apple juice.
• Green tea with lemon.

After you consume your morning tonic, try to include a minimum of two servings of food choices from each of the Tropical Diet Detox food groups listed in the table on page 34 throughout the day. Organic is the best choice. Fresh comes next followed by frozen or canned as long as it's low-sodium, sugar-free, and fat-free.

The foods can be eaten raw, steamed, or pureed. Fried, grilled, or sautéed are not suggested during the initial phase. If you are unfamiliar with the food item or recipe, the food and recipe guide is listed at the end of the chapter or in Appendix A.

To enhance the taste and detoxing action of your diet, use the herbs to flavor each meal. This will be especially helpful if you choose to consume the same diet daily.

No other foods, herbs, or salt are permitted on this phase of the program unless a physical condition or illness requires you to do so.

Tropical Diet Phase-One Detox Food Groups and Servings®

Food Group	Pro (Gms)	Carb (Gms)	Fat (Gms)	Energy (Calorie) Levels* 1200 Detox—women	1500 Detox—men
Milk or Milk Substitutes 100 calories/serving soy rice based milk, yogurt, frozen yogurt—no sugar	8	12	varies 1	1-soy, rice based	2-soy, rice based
Fruit **60 calories/serving** berries, mango, kiwi, pineapple, guava, lychee, carambola, passion fruit, mamey		15		6	6
Vegetables **50 calories/cup** sprouts, broccoli, onions, peppers, chayote, asparagus, mushrooms, cabbage, chili, chives, garlic, okra, kale, lettuce, spinach	4	10	varies	3 cups+	3 cups+
Grains/Starches **80 calories/serving-** **¼-½ cup** calabaza, cassava, rice, potato, legume, beans, rice crackers pasta-legume, potato or rice based, pupadims, peas, sweet potato, spaghetti squash jackfruit/breadfruit	3	15	varies	4	4
Protein/Meat Substitutes **55-75 cal/oz** fish-salmon, tuna, sardines, bluefish, mackerel, conch, dolphin, mahi mahi & egg whites (5=1 oz. pro)	7-10	0	varies	8 oz. or equiv	9 oz. or equiv
Fat- **45 calories/serving-1 tsp** Seeds, nuts, dressing olive oil, flax, avocado, almonds		5		3	4
Total Calories*: **Grams (g)/Percent% calories from:**				1200 cal	1525 cal
Carbohydrates **Protein** **Fat**				162 g (54%) 82 g (27%) 25 g (19%)	204 g (54%) 103 g (27%) 33 g (19%)

Table 2
Tropical Diet Detox Food and Herb Groups

Gastrointestinal Stimulation	Fluid Elimination	Blood Purification
apples	apples	garlic
cucumber	cucumber	leek
onion	onion	onion
artichokes	asparagus	essential fatty acids
beets	mushrooms	omega-3s in ground
cruciferous vegetables:	parsley	flax and fish oil
cabbage, broccoli	tarragon	
cauliflower,		
brussels sprouts		
kale		
onions and garlic		
ground flaxseed		
olive oil (no more than 3 tsp. daily)		

Circulation	Perspiration
fresh ginger	garlic
oregano	onion
rosemary	chives
cayenne	chile peppers
	mustard
	green tea
	thyme

Vegetable Tian
SERVES: 1

A detox recipe appetizer, or main course served with soup and salad. Adapted from a Chef Lee Goble recipe.

Ingredients:

2 oz. bok choy leaves	1 fl oz. Balsamic vinegar
½ oz. Carrot	½ oz. Tomato
½ oz. Leek	½ oz. Mushroom
½ oz. Celery	
½ oz. Peppers	• ¼ tsp Olive oil

Procedure:

1. Chop ingredients into attractive slivers. Sautee with vinegar.
2. Soften bok choy leafs until tender but not fragile.
3. Wrap ingredients into tight rolls.
4. Bathe in olive oil to seal.
5. Garnish with shredded carrots.

Substitutions:

- Any green leaves will work for wrapping. You can even use sushi wrap.
- Any combination of fresh vegetables will work. Follow portion size and variety of colors.
- Any vinegar including rice, raspberry, or other flavors will work.
- Any flavored olive oil will work. Any unsaturated oil will work for post-Detox phase meal plans.

Tropical Diet Food Servings: 1 c vegetables, 1 fat

End-of-the-Chapter Questions

1. WHAT IS A THE TROPICAL DIET DETOX?

The Tropical Diet Detox is an elimination program, i.e., removal of poor food choices, eating habits, food obsessions and compulsions, stagnant exercise programs, and unhealthy lifestyle choices like late nights, smoking, and excessive intakes of alcohol and drugs in your life which sabotage your efforts to permanently change your behavior and prevent long-term weight loss, overall health, and peak performance in sports, health, and in life.

2. WHO SHOULD START A DETOX PROGRAM?

Anyone who plans on completing a successful Tropical Diet experience for weight loss, overall health and energy levels, and for sports performance. It can also benefit those with a score of more than 10 on the Detox Assessment located at the beginning of the chapter.

3. WHERE IS THE BEST PLACE AND TIME TO START THE TROPICAL DIET DETOX PROGRAM?

Ideally, the best place to start the program is in the privacy of your home, in a quiet vacation spot, and while on a personal break from work and family responsibilities.

4. HOW LONG SHOULD I STAY ON THE TROPICAL DIET DETOX PROGRAM?

The Detox phase of the Tropical Diet can take as little as a day and up to two weeks. It all depends on the amount and intensity of dietary and behavioral vices you have. If you're planning on giving up dairy it could take a day. Something like alcohol can take several days before withdrawal symptoms are complete.

Since it takes the gastrointestinal tract three days to turn over, you should ideally plan on a minimum of a three-day period. It takes much longer for your brain and behaviors to catch up—often up to 8 weeks.

5. WHAT TYPE OF FOOD, EATING, AND BEHAVIORAL VICES SHOULD BE ELIMINATED DURING THE TROPICAL DIET EATING PROGRAM?

There are dozens of appropriate foods for detoxing. Check the list on pages 33 to 34.

6. WHAT ABOUT EXERCISE?

Exercise assists the detox process by speeding up the clearance of toxins through your body. You'll notice changes in your appearance, physical, mental, and spiritual well-being almost immediately because exercising encourages healthy circulation and elimination.

Any exercise that causes you to sweat for a minimum of 30 minutes each day, such as stretching, Pilates, yoga, walking, cycling, or jogging will assist your detox by increasing the following:

- Breathing and sweating.
- Lymph flow to create urine.
- Bowel movements.
- Blood circulation and turnover.
- Liver action.
- Sweating and exhalation.

You can start a mild stretching program or a walking program for 30 minutes each day. After you master the stretching and walking program, you can progress to other forms of exercise such as jogging, cycling, swimming, yoga, or Pilates.

However, it is best not to start a new, rigorous exercise program without your physician's approval especially if you are older than 40 years old or have a previous medical condition which compromises your ability to work out.

If you want to add an additional detox aid, head to your local spa or resort and see a licensed therapist for a massage, body scrub, and/or detox wrap. All of these therapeutic rubs will assist your body in moving out the toxins and get your body going even when it's not doing so by itself.

And if you can't afford to get to a spa, there are a number of detox scrubs and masks available at your local pharmacy, beauty salon, or department store. Try to get the most natural products available, made without perfumes or animal testing.

7. HOW WILL I KNOW IF I HAVE BEEN SUCCESSFUL WITH MY DETOX?

You will know you are successful with the detox when you no longer feel withdrawal symptoms such as headaches, dizziness, nausea, cravings, and/or obsessions to shop, buy, or stock your personal poison in your home or office. You may still think about your favorite toxins but do not have the urge to purchase them and destroy your progress.

One place you may find detox success is in the privacy of your bathroom. Are you ready? Here goes.

Look in the toilet after you urinate. If your urine is a dark yellow color or even a brownish tint you may be dehydrated. It's a good signal to drink more water on your program. Up to eight cups are recommended each day. If your urine is clear, you are in the clear and are probably not dehydrated. Smelly urine means you may be continuing to pass toxins, although some of the detox foods like asparagus, onions, garlic, and beets can leave a foul odor in your urine.

This also applies to bowel movements. If you are constipated, it may mean you need to eat more high-fiber foods from the list, and drink more water or detox tonics. If you are consuming too much fiber and going to the bathroom more than three times a day, you may want to add a cup of cooked brown rice with your vegetables and cut back on the amount of vegetables and fruits you are consuming. If the stools are pure liquid or the diet causes you to have an urgency to defecate, you need to pull back immediately and speak with your physician.

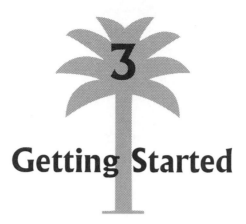

Getting Started

How to Use the Program

Pack your bags, it's time to leave for your Tropical Dietary vacation. The surf is up, the sun is shining bright and your cocoa-buttered, dark handsome lover is waiting for you to slip into your bathing suit and share a cool, refreshing drink.

Preparing for this diet is as fun and easy as getting ready for an island adventure. Let's get this party started.

Level One—The Detox

DAYS 1 TO 3

You've already had a chance to take the plunge and detox from all your vices in Chapter 2. If you've chosen to move onto the *L.A.B.* plan in the next section of this chapter then go ahead and take your Tropical Diet Taste Test at this time.

If you are hesitant to move on without at least one mini-detox, then stay with me here. These first three days of The Tropical Diet could also be well spent focusing on the ground level of the Food, Fitness, and Pleasure Pyramid© described in Chapter 1. This is actually the best time to enhance your awareness of the world around you so you can appreciate your dietary vacation even more. Take a deep breath, have a cool drink, and find a physical activity that makes you sweat, feel, or touch someone you love.

BUYER BEWARE

If you chose to skip this part and get started on your *L.A.B.* plan immediately, think again. Detoxing is your prerequisite to permanent change, confessing your dietary sins, and committing to a healthy future. However, pick your battles wisely. I realize you might not want to give up all your vices right away. It's almost unrealistic and impossible to do all at once. Just keep in mind, you can always revisit this step in four weeks and start fresh with an even better detox goal in mind.

Level Two—Nourishing your Body with Energy-Building Nutrients

DAYS 4 TO 7

Now that you've established your long-term goals and you're ready to get this dietary vacation started, you can move onto the next level of Tropical Dieting. First take your Tropical Diet Taste Test on page 63 so you know which plan you will be following. A description of each of the *L*ean, *A*thlete, and *B*asic plans can be found starting on page 75.

After you have found the best plan for you, select any healthy food choices from the Tropical Diet Foundation food lists on pages 133 to 141, but I have a few house rules for getting started.

Here goes.

- Limit your food choices to five foods from each of The Tropical Diet Food Groups: protein, starch, vegetables, fruits, dairy equivalents, and fats. The most nutritious food choices can be found on the food lists, menus, and also highlighted in the Nutrition Nugget charts located throughout the book. However you may also feel free to choose your personal favorites from each of the food groups as long as you can control the portion sizes to reach 1,500 calories for men and 1,200 calories for women.

Limiting your food choices for the first week or two will minimize the anxiety associated with dieting and will allow you to concentrate on other important everyday life issues such as family and work rather than your food choices and preparation.

• Eat foods like salad, soup, and consommés, and drink tea or coffee before your meals when possible.
This will help you to fill up and reduce your total calorie intake at mealtime.

• Eat in one specific location, e.g., the kitchen table, the office lunchroom.
This will help you to modify your eating behaviors and train you for better behaviors whether you're eating an apple or apple pie.

• Update your Tropical Diet Pocket Coach© food record (available at the website) before or during the meal.
This will help you to commit, confess, and control your total calorie intake.

• Drink a minimum of 1 cup of water, tea, or sparkling water ½ hour before mealtime.
This will help keep you hydrated and will help you determine your actual versus perceived hunger level. Hunger often masks dehydration.

• Make sure your meal includes one raw food which requires chewing, e.g., carrot, celery, jicama, or red pepper sticks.
These foods will exercise your face muscles and your mind and help satiate your appetite than if you only selected easy-to-eat foods like mashed potatoes, or cereal and milk.

• Include a tropically filling fruit with nonfat yogurt dip for dessert. Eat orange, grapefruit, kiwi, and/or pineapple slices, a whole apple or pear upon meal completion.
Eating these foods is more nutritious than empty-calorie desserts and a great sugar substitute.

Research has shown that these tips will help you become a successful calorie-controlled eater naturally and for life.

During week one, it's also time to explore the complete Tropical Diet Food Lists including the Tropical Kitchen staple list and menus on page 128 to 169 so you can get a head start on your *L.A.B.* program for the weeks to come. Study the serving sizes of your favorite foods, or even new foods on your lists to familiarize yourself with the varying portion sizes of foods according to their calorie, carbohydrate, protein, and fat contents.

It's an ideal time to get *Supermarket Savvy*©, the buzz trade newsletter (see appendix) which you can order to find out the latest supermarket trends, new food items and reviews of new food items already at your grocery store. Learn to read the information on food labels. Apply the calories, grams of carbohydrates, proteins, and fats to your *L.A.B.* plan to see how any food can fit into your program. And check out the glossary. Find out about all the delicious and exotic tropically nutritious foods just waiting for you to prepare and bite into them.

As you get carried away in your dietary adventure, just don't forget to keep track of what you eat in your Tropical Diet Pocket Coach© pads. This is really the best way to control your dietary intake regardless of your plan, calorie needs, and unexpected adventures to parties, social events, and business get-togethers.

And finally, week one is a great time to touch base with your Tropical Diet Nutritionist if you run into a snag or have a question. No matter how simple or stupid the question may seem to you, we are here to answer your email or phone calls so don't hesitate. Better to be nutritionally safe than sorry.

Level Three—Shake Your Booty

INCORPORATE ANYTHING THAT MAKES YOU SWEAT

During weeks one to two, it's also time to shake your booty and work up a sweat. Not only will you get into better shape, burn more calories, and just feel better, you can also earn Tropical Bonus Points for your exercise program. Since exercise is one of the most important aspects to long-term weight management, and yes, since it does burn extra fat calories for you, you can even eat some extra calories above and beyond your *L.A.B.* prescription.

The Tropical Diet Bonus Points reward you for your efforts by giving you extra food calories to spend each day. This means for every hour of exercise, you get to include additional calories above and beyond your dietary program. The chart below summarizes your bonus calories for exercise.

Exercise Bonus Chart

If you:	Then you may add an additional:
Perform light exercise—stretching, yoga, Pilates, walking 30 minutes each day	100 calories of approved food each day
Work out your heart 1 hour each day with swimming, jogging, walking (4 miles/ hour or faster), cycling, dancing, or spinning	200 calories of approved foods each day
Work your heart with a 1-hour session, each morning and do strength training at least 3 times each week	200 calories approved foods plus a 200 cal free snack, your choice of food or beverage each day

If you're uncomfortable adding calories and would rather lose weight faster, try this.

Add a new exercise or routine that includes an island beat. It could be a salsa or calypso dance class, Rasta yoga (I found this at Sandals Grande in Ocho Rios, Jamaica, and it was fabulous), water Pilates, or water spinning class. There are also U.S. Swimming Master swimming classes offered by many clubs, universities, and local schools to help older swimmers brush up on their strokes, kicks, and overall swim skills. Swimming will also get you into a bathing suit regardless of the season or climate where you live.

You can even try something really different like training for a marathon. *Team in Training*™, a program designed to match primarily first-time marathoners with cancer patients provides coaching and travel stipends for those who raise money for the Leukemia Society.

Millions of runners have been born this way, and dollars have been raised for research and recovery needs.

You can train for fun "musically themed" marathons or half-marathons such as the Rock n' Roll Marathon in California; Arizona, Virginia, and Tennessee. Some of my personal favorites include the Disney World Marathon in Orlando, Florida; Big Sur Marathon in Carmel, California or Marine Corps Marathon in Washington, D.C. If you prefer a tropical venue, there are several marathons that will accommodate your desire. There is Negril, Jamaica's Reggae Marathon; Bermuda, Tahiti, or the Maui Marathons, too.

If there is one thing I want you to know about the best exercise program it is to find the exercise you like and to stick with it once you do. Exercise is one of the key aspects of successful weight loss programs regardless of the original weight loss diet.

Level Four

WEEKS 3 TO 4

Time to get this Food Fitness™ vacation going.

Take the program up a notch on the Food, Fitness, and Pleasure Pyramid© and try a tempting taste, something tasty, something spicy or exotic, like a sassy island spice, ethnic food, or seasoning that you've never tried before. It's like a long-standing relationship. You look for new perfumes, hairstyles, or lingerie to spice things up. Well, it's the same with your Tropical Diet.

Now, I want you to consider something radical.

Get in the car and head to the grocery and select at least one new food and maybe even a few new foods to add to your diet. Look for tropical flavors, colors, and tastes and treat yourself to some of the delicious recipes throughout the book. You may select from gourmet cuisine or *"convenience cuisine"* (see page 157 to 163) depending on your time factor. And if you don't have the time to cook, don't sweat over it. Save the sweat for something else like a good workout.

It may also be a good time to head out to a Latin, Caribbean, Asian-style, or New World cuisine restaurant which features The Tropical Diet cuisine. A listing of the Tropical Diet—friendly restaurants is located at *www.thetropicaldiet.com* website.

If you're not comfortable stepping out just yet, stick to your five food choices from each group, each day, however, try this: Hop over to the ethnic food section of your grocery store and try a fresh new spice like ginger or cilantro, seasoning like Jamaican jerk seasoning or even chili sauce to dress up your appetizer, salad, main course, or side dish.

You can also vary the cut of meat, poultry, or fish you normally consume. Try something new like game, veal, duck or lamb, and season it with the tropical seasonings you purchase.

Who knows?

By coincidence, you may even add a missing nutrient to your diet or increase the amount of calories your body burns with some of the hotter ingredients like hot pepper, chili sauce, and chili peppers.

Level Five—Comfort Yourself with Something Sweet and Satisfying, Cool and Refreshing

WEEK 4 TO 5

Did you know it's actually good to cheat on your diet?

Yes, once in a while, it helps your body to increase its calorie intake, change the carbohydrate protein or fat composition, decrease or increase your exercise level to wake up the system. Research suggests change is good, especially while dieting. So go for it!

So it's time to take a break and really enjoy this dietary vacation. It's a built-in binge so take advantage of it. You've worked hard for three weeks so it's time for to comfort yourself with your favorite food or beverage. You've been disciplined on the program for 21 days so it's time to celebrate on your terms. Don't wait until you're out of control to indulge in your favorite food fantasy.

Have a tropical martini or a frozen pina colada. Share a fresh slice of key lime pie with someone you love. Live a little.

The best way to plan for this dietary break is to make the "switch"— change your *L.A.B.* prescription to one of the other plans so you can accommodate your sweet, meaty, or refreshing indulgence. So even if you choose the same calorie level, change the food program like this.

For example, if you would like to have something sweet or high in carbohydrates switch from the *L*ean to the *A*thlete's program for a day.

If you're an athlete who would like to indulge in a thick and juicy 16-ouncer, switch to the *L*ean or *B*asic program.

And, if you've been balancing your protein, carbohydrates, and fats at every meal for all this time on the *B*asic plan, take a break. Enjoy the *L*ean or *A*thlete's plan for a day or two.

The key to making a successful switch is to:

- Continue on your *L.A.B.* calorie prescription.
- Add additional exercise time to your current regime.
- Leave the guilt behind. Everyone deserves a free day from time to time even when dieting for weight loss, health, or training. RELAX!

Tomorrow, you can start your four-week cycle all over again.

Level Six

NUTRITIONAL ENLIGHTENMENT

At this point, you've probably lost anywhere from 5 to 15 pounds, or several inches and some body fat. You feel and look good. You're energized, healthier, and happy with your accomplishment. This is the same kind of feeling you get when you graduate from high school, receive a promotion at work, or even after a fabulous tropical vacation. This feeling or euphoria, I placed at the peak of the Food, Fitness, and Pleasure Pyramid©. This is the top level you can climb for now, the highest state of consciousness. Abraham Maslow, a well-known social psychologist referred to this peak in emotional life and called it self-actualization.

The Tropical Diet actually helps you to self-actualize, nutritionally. You have learned how to breathe, sweat, and eat healthy. You've tried new foods, a variety of ethnic cuisines, spices, or dance classes and have familiarized yourself with at least one tropical or ethnic food. You now exercise on a regular basis. You've even learned how to get loose enjoying an occasional frozen fruit drink, delicious dessert, or even a calypso night on the town. You have earned the right to feel good about yourself. It was hard work but you made it.

Now, its time to reevaluate your program goals. If you still need to lose some weight, reduce your cholesterol levels, or train for your favorite sport you can continue on your same *L.A.B.* plan or reevaluate the need for a new program with your Tropical Diet Nutritionist. If you don't need to lose weight, it's time to learn how to maintain your terrific weight and fat loss.

Either way, the honeymoon is over but not your lust and love for life, good food, and good health. However, now comes the hard part. In order to keep the magic in this dietary relationship going, there are a few tricks of the trade you can use. Here they are.

The key to long-term success is:

- To continually set new goals for you. These may or may not include weight goals. Life is a continuous cycle. Keep the fire and energy going by looking for something special to shoot for.
- Include a new exercise routine or class. Sweating with others is *sexy*.
- Train for a triathlon—a swim, bike, and run competition of varying distances. It's fun, refreshing, and exciting. Almost anyone at any age can give it a try.
- Take your mate to a new restaurant which features Tropical Diet cuisine. A romantic evening without the dietary guilt!
- Shop at an ethnic or gourmet market and explore new ingredients, foods, or products. It's much more fun than your neighborhood grocery store.
- Start saving up for an exotic tropical vacation like those I've highlighted at my website or in this book. For every calorie you've burned for exercise or saved by selecting healthier food choices, save a buck. Just think, you'll be flying off in no time at all!

End-of-the-Chapter Questions:

1. HOW CAN YOU LOSE WEIGHT AND MAINTAIN YOUR ENERGY LEVELS AT THE SAME TIME WHILE FOLLOWING THE TROPICAL DIET?

Energy is the way to describe your body's capacity to do anything you like to do, whether it's work, compete at your favorite sport, or play with your dog at the park. The sun is our ultimate energy source. Through a process called photosynthesis, the sun passes its energy onto green plants through sunlight. The sun's rays then penetrate the plant's chemical bonds to provide "energy" in the form of glucose, commonly known as sugar. This is the first and most basic energy step.

From this simplest form of sugar, proteins, fats, and other sugars (carbohydrates) are created. Animals and humans get these energy sources through food. The Tropical Diet translates this scientific energy formula into nutritious, cost-effective, naturally portion-sized energy sources on your *L*ean, *A*thlete, or *B*asic food plans (Chapters 5 to 7).

2. HOW MANY CALORIES DO I NEED TO EAT EACH DAY TO GET ENOUGH ENERGY?

Each one of us has our own personal best energy prescription. Too many or too few calories will cause you to lose or gain too much weight. Therefore, calculating your energy prescription is an important step towards successful lifelong weight and energy management.

Three factors influence your daily personal calorie needs. They are the:

• **Basal Metabolic Rate (BMR):** the minimal amount of calories required to sustain all the body's normal functions such as breathing, digesting and metabolizing foods, and eliminating waste products. The BMR represents 60 to 70% of calories needed for Total Energy Expenditure (TEE). Of this:

—29% is used by the liver for making glucose (sugars) and ketones bodies for the brain.

— 19% for the brain.

— 18% for resting muscles.

— 10% for the heart.

— 7% for the kidney, and

— 17% for the remainder of the organs.

• **Energy Expended for Physical Activity (EEPA):** includes exercise and everyday activities like mowing the lawn or washing the dishes (see Table 3). For couch potatoes, this can account for 100 calories each day. For athletes, it can run as high as double the amount of your basal calories expended for training each day.

• **Thermic Effect of Food (TEF)** aka known as Specific Dynamic Action (SDA) of food. Accounts for the amount of energy required to digest and metabolize food. It is approximately 10% of the sum, of the basal metabolic calories and activity (BMR+EEPE) calories added together.

Your Energy Prescription

There are many methods for calculating your personal BMR but I will leave the more complicated methods for the athlete's section in Chapter 5. For now, all you need to know is the simplest method to calculate your daily minimal calorie needs.

Follow along with me. Just take your desirable body weight in pounds and multiply that number by 10 calories per pound. That means if you would like to weigh 125 pounds, your BMR would be 125 x 10 calories which comes to 1,250 calories a day. If you want to weight 180 your BMR calories would be 1,800 calories.

After calculating your minimal calorie needs, you can skip over to Chapter 3 and get started right away on your personal Tropical Diet Plan. Just take the amount of calories you just calculated, take the Tropical Diet Taste Test and choose the appropriate calorie level of the ℒean, 𝒜thlete, or ℬasic plan. If you want to be more precise about your daily calorie needs, continue along in this chapter, and you'll learn how to add additional calories for exercise and for digestive calorie needs (SDA).

> ### Formula for BMR
>
> Desired weight x 10 calories per pound.
> If you want to weigh 125 then multiply it by 10 calories. This will give you
> 1,250 calories. Take the Taste Test (page 63) and choose the 1,200 calorie
> Tropical Diet *L.A.B.* plans which is best for you.

3. WHAT FACTORS AFFECT THE RATE MY BODY USES CALORIES?

Your personal basal metabolic rate can be as low as 1,000 calories or as high as 2,500 calories depending on your desirable body weight, age, and gender and health status. Other factors also affect your BMR. Hereditary alone may account for a 40% variation in BMR between individuals. This is why you may know someone your size, height, and weight who can eat whatever they want and never gain weight.

Other factors listed on the following chart.

Factors Which May Affect BMR Calories

Age	The younger you are, the more calories you use. You lose 2 to 3% of your total BMR calories each decade after 18 years old. That means you'll need to cut out about 100 to 200 calories of carbohydrate containing foods each decade if you want to try to remain the same weight throughout your lifetime.
Gender	Women have 5 to 10% lower metabolic rates than men even if they are the same size and weight, the good news? The menstrual cycle increases your BMR by approximately 150 calories a day during the second half of the menstrual cycle.
Growth	Children and pregnant women have higher BMR rates.
Body composition	More muscle means more calories used at rest.
Fever	Fever raises BMR by 7% for each degree above 98.6° F.
Stress	Stress hormones raise the BMR.

Environmental

Temperature	Cold and heat raise BMR; if you live in the tropics, you have a 5 to 20% higher BMR than those living in more temperate areas. Exercising in rooms or weather above 86 degrees also increases the caloric expenditure by 5% from sweating. Exercising in cold weather depends on the clothing worn and the individual's percent body fat.
Fasting/Starvation	Lowers the BMR
Malnutrition	Poor eating habits lower the BMR
Thyroid hormone	Thyroxine controls the internal calorie regulator; if you have less thyroxine (determined by a blood test) you will have a slower metabolism.
Thermic affect of food	In leaner people, energy speeds up after consuming food, while in the obese, no change occurs.

4. HOW CAN I JUMPSTART MY METABOLISM IF IT IS NATU-RALLY SLUGGISH FROM DIETING OR BECOMES SLUGGISH WHILE FOLLOWING THIS PROGRAM?

There are three ways that you can kick up your metabolism. I can sum up this answer with a short discussion on food, fitness, and mind metabolics. These are the only ways you can speed up your metabolism naturally, without the use of diet pills, energy drinks, or drugs. This section shows you the fitness routines and mental metabolism techniques which will rev up the way your body uses food calories and mentally move the calories out for the ultimate body burn.

Exercise . . .

is not a four letter word.

It's the best way to change how your body uses calories and to speed up your metabolism so you either lose weight faster or tolerate more food each day. Any exercise or activity will do. The beauty is that exercise increases your body's basal calorie needs up to 500%. How?

Exercise helps your body to use more calories by increasing:

- Muscle mass, and lean body mass, and decreasing fat.
- The amount of calories you expend or use each day.
- The calories you use for eating, digestion, and post-meal calorie expenditure.
- The amount of fat your body uses for ordinary activities throughout the day.

And by improving:

• Your personal perception, self-esteem, mood, and body image so you move better, use more energy for sitting and standing, speaking, and work:
• Your sleep which has been shown to improve daily calorie expenditure, recovery, and rest so you can start all over again the following day.

Here are ten of the easiest ways to sneak a workout into your daily routine:

1. Start the day with a stretch in bed, walk with your pet, or jog to get the morning newspaper.
2. Take the steps whenever you can: at the mall, work, or your children's school.
3. Turn on MTV or your favorite radio station and blast it. You're likely to shake your booty harder and enjoy your house chores with a little background rhythm.
4. Do push-ups between vacuuming each room, dusting each table, or mopping each floor.
5. Take a walk after you drop off the kids at school. Instead of fighting traffic, take a 20-minute jaunt to burn some fat and release those endorphins, the chemicals which will prepare you to handle a stressful day at work.
6. Wear a 10-pound to 15-pound vest when you clean the house to boost the calorie burn of vacuuming, dusting, or mopping.
7. Mix in a dose of heavy cleaning each day such as scrubbing, or carrying heavy items, such as laundry baskets up and down steps.
8. Pace while you speak on the telephone.
9. Stand while you use the computer. Standing for an hour each day will burn an extra 5,000 to 7,000 calories each year.
10. Walk from room to room to communicate to family members instead of shouting or using an intercom.

And since we know from the *Weight Registry* that people who walk about 4 miles each day are more successful at long-term weight loss, try these activities if you're not up to walking each day to get a similar effect:

Mile Equivalents for a Variety of Activities

Activity	Minutes per One Mile
Baseball/Softball	
Fielder	28
Pitcher	19
Basketball	12
Calisthenics: sit-ups, push-ups	25
Circuit Training	15
Dancing	17
Gardening:	
Digging	11
Hedging	22
Mowing	15
Raking	32
Golf	20
Hiking	20
Jumping Rope	11
Karate	9
Rowing	12
Stair Climbing	8
Tennis	14
Weight Training	14

Adapted from the American Running and Fitness Organization Exercise across America Chart

Mental Metabolism

The mind is a strong and powerful organ, probably the most influential factor in determining how much exercise you will do, how many calories you use each day, and ultimately your motivation for continuing on your personal diet program.

Think of it this way.

It takes an enormous amount of effort just to get out of bed each day. Imagine if you used the same kind of energy to avoid dietary pitfalls like:

- Food shopping when hungry.
- Eating when stressed.
- Purchasing foods in bulk.
- Buying personal "binge" foods to stock for a "bad" day at work.

- Eating at the computer, your work desk, in front of the TV, standing up with an open fridge door, in the car, or on the run.
- Drinking cocktails or going to a cocktail party on an empty stomach.
- Eating without accountability—not taking stock and control of your portion sizes or overall food intake.
- Eating as a reward to losing weight!

So how do you keep up the momentum with your diet so you reach your personal goal weight and health goals?

There are many ways. Here are some of the best:

- Find a dietary soul mate. You can enlist the help of your lover, spouse, friend, neighbor, children, spiritual leader, or even your pet. Yes, even pets can be therapeutic when it comes to assisting with the exercise and eating plan. Just take a look at the exercise and eating patterns of a cat or a bird and take some notes!
- Find a training partner at work, through your local sports magazine, community fitness club, Y, or church/temple to meet on an ongoing basis for exercise, eating, or discussion (in that order).
- Hire a nutrition expert, a registered dietitian (RD), to help establish your Tropical Diet program and goals and assist you along the way. The names of RD referrals can be found at *www.thetropicaldiet.com* website.
- Make your house Tropical Diet–friendly. Purchase the foundation foods on pages 133 to 141. To play it safe, get rid of the foods that sabotage your efforts. There are millions of hungry and homeless people in this country. Give it away!
- Try one new Tropical Diet food selection each week. Liven and excite your senses and stimulate your healthy eating appetite with some fun foods found on the best snack choices and author's select food choices.
- Take your measurements and pictures of yourself as you're losing the weight fat and inches. Don't rely on the scale. The pounds will fall off as you adapt new foods, exercise, and rev up your mind.
- Buy a tropical fitness outfit, bathing suit, or exercise outfit that accents your best features. If you have blue eyes, go for color. If you have a slim waist, show it off. If your arms look pumped let

the world know about them in a sleeveless tropical color tank. Reinforce your look with bright energetic clothes. Brighten up your old wardrobe with new fashions. You don't need to spend a lot of money. My favorite places to shop are at closeouts, secondhand or vintage shops, and online.

And when you hit a weight plateau . . .

When your metabolism is stuck in a rut, you can actually change and readjust the way your body uses calories. Here are 10 simple adjustments you can make to your food choices, meal timing, exercise, and mental approach that can rev up the rate of your body's burning capabilities.

---

10 Ways to Boost your Metabolism

1. Eat several meals and snacks each day.
2. Get moving! Build muscle through any type of exercise from active house-keeping and scrubbing to jogging. Anything will do. And if you're a veteran exerciser, vary what you do by trying something new. If you're a runner, add cycling, swimming, or Pilates. If you are a yoga junkie, try a long walk or weight training.
3. Add chili pepper, a hot spice, or hot sauce to some of your favorite dishes. The capsaicin will rev up your metabolism.
4. Add protein, especially at breakfast and dinner. Protein has a higher rate of calorie burn than carbohydrates and fat.
5. Try a tropically healthy high-fiber food. The fiber will rev up your digestional metabolism.
6. Breathe. The deeper you breathe, the more you will send messages to your cells to use fat for energy
7. Think like a fast-moving person even if you're not. Translate your mind speed into body speed.
8. Add a cup of java, tea, or caffeine-rich beverage every few hours if you're in good health and your personal physician approves this dietary change.
9. Meet and eat your BEE daily calorie needs.
10. Make the "switch"! Change you're eating plan every 5th day. Surprise your body with the *Lean* plan if you're following the *Athlete's* plan; switch to the Basic plan if you're following the *Lean* plan and take a day off from the *Athlete's* plan and switch to the *Lean* or *Basic* plan. The *switch* will surprise your body with a different set of nutrients to process and keep your system on its toes!

On a final metabolic note, since your body is always evolving, it's important to get a metabolic "check-up" at least once a year. Check with your doctor (MD) about taking a blood test to assess your thyroid hormones, the body's metabolic regulators. Make sure you also have your cholesterol, blood fats, and complete blood count checked at the same time.

Then speak to your registered dietitian (RD) and get the best diet for your health and metabolic needs. You can always pick up your Tropical Diet Book or email your Tropical Diet Nutritionist to get your best program and start your program all over again.

THE TROPICAL DIET
L.A.B.

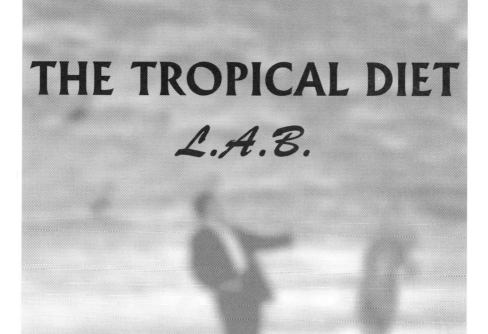

Part II

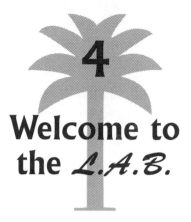

Welcome to
the *L.A.B.*

Just imagine yourself in the middle of the Caribbean island lounging on your own beach with someone you love. Between your pearl white recliners, there is a table with cocktail size seafood bites, bright crisp vegetables with dip, juicy sliced pineapple, kiwi and strawberries and a bubbling glass of champagne. Waiting on a boat offshore is your main course of grilled meats, pan-fried fish and stir-fried vegetables. Dessert is just a boat ride away.

And guess what. Your Tropical Diet personalized program includes all of these foods and much more.

You see, there are no perfect foods, no perfect diet.

No One Diet Fits All

Medical and nutrition experts agree that no superior weight control program works better over another when it comes to permanent weight loss. In fact, only 5% of dieters keep the weight off in the long run. Researchers from The University of Pennsylvania School of Medicine recently confirmed this when they compared the success rates of four programs: Atkins, Dean Ornish, Weight Watchers, and the Zone (40/30/30) regimens. In a year, participants lost only 5% of their original body weight. However, all the programs helped to decease their risk for heart disease by 7 to 15%. Another classic study confirmed that regardless of carbohydrate diets varying from 25%, 45%, or 75% on a 1,200 calorie diet all of the regimens proved to be equally as successful in weight loss efforts.

Bottom line.

The ultimate goal of any diet is to assist the estimated 54 million American dieters to lose excess body fat by providing a healthy, tasty, and attractive eating program and help them to stay healthy, energized, and satisfied with their food choices. The program that contains all the ingredients of the successful weight loss recipe is The Tropical Diet.

Experts agree that regardless of the dieter's program choice, the weight loss plan must include specific nutritional and behavioral components. Most of the passing diet fads are either deficient in calories, vitamins, minerals, protein, carbohydrates, and/or fiber. Some of the diets can lead to dietary deficiencies if they were followed for any great length of time. Many set the dieter up for fast results, unrealistic expectations, guilt, a feeling of helplessness, and failure.

So why are fad diets so attractive to millions of dieters each year? Here's why:

- Fad diets offer a quick-fix mentality guaranteeing instant results.
- Dieters prefer to eat a lot of one food group, i.e. proteins, fruits, and have trouble with the moderation mantra.
- While the jury is still out on the perfect diet within the nutrition and medical communities, legitimate or not, the non-credentialed diet book authors tend to be dramatic and convincing.
- Appearance is a more powerful motivator than health and weight responsibility. Dieters want to look good fast regardless of the health implications.

Experts have looked at the popular diet issue to assess the efficacy of their weight loss and maintenance, effect on metabolism, psychological well-being, and disease risk reduction premise.

A summary of these results concluded that[1]:

- Low-carbohydrate diets like *Atkins*® and *The Carbohydrate Addicts Diet* which provide less than 20% (100 grams) carbs and 55 to 65% fat, suppress appetite to only a small degree and produce a very rapid weight loss from diuresis.
- Zone type diets with 40% dietary carbohydrates and a balance of 30% from carbohydrates and protein encourage weight loss via low calories and not from the magic it claims to have on managing blood sugars.
- Very low-fat diets such as Dr. Dean Ornish and the Pritikin program, encourage rapid weight loss but tend to be very restrictive with animal products.

Successful weight loss depends on many factors. Experts agree that obesity is a chronic condition that cannot be treated for a few months with a strenuous diet[2]. Weight control must be a lifelong effort of adhering to a safe and effective plan. The following elements need to be highlighted with any weight loss plan:

- Include all of the RDAs for vitamins, minerals, and protein.
- Low in calories not in nutritional value.
- Directed towards a slow and steady weight loss, about a pound a week.

Welcome to the $\mathcal{L}.\mathcal{A}.\mathcal{B}.$

The nutritional composition of your diet absolutely plays a key role in your weight loss success.

The Tropical Diet uses the latest medical research to apply the principles of food analysis, metabolism and appetite and combines this information with sound nutrition principles for the $\mathcal{L}$ean, $\mathcal{A}$thletic and, $\mathcal{B}$asic ($\mathcal{L}.\mathcal{A}.\mathcal{B}.$) plans for your Tropical Diet program.

This chapter describes your $\mathcal{L}.\mathcal{A}.\mathcal{B}.$ plans, benefits, controversies, and challenges, food choices and menus for each of the programs. The major difference between each plan is the percentage of carbohydrate, protein and fat of the diet.

---

1 The U.S. Department of Agricultural Research Education and Economics
2 US Department of Health and Human Services of the National Institutes of Health (NIH.)

WHICH DIET IS FOR YOU?

The best *L.A.B.* plan for you is the one that is determined from the results from the Tropical Diet Taste Test on the following page. The Tropical Diet Taste Test was developed to help you select your best eating program based on your lifestyle, personal preferences, and factors which can make the difference between success and failure on a nutritional program.

Regardless of the results from the Taste Test, ultimately, the eating plan that will work best for you will:

• Help you lose weight fast and safely.
• Without leaving you hungry after meals.
• And will energize you throughout the day.

Before you get started, there's probably a few terms you need to know.

Sugar-sensitive: Mood and energy levels affected by sugar intake without a clinical problem such as diabetes or hypoglycemia.

Satiation: Feeling of fullness or gratification of appetite.

Metabolism: the sum of all chemical changes in the body.

Plateau: a normal part of weight loss when your body is adjusting to lower calories and stops losing weight.

Syndrome X: a cluster of four symptoms including diabetes, abnormal blood lipid levels, high blood pressure and obesity which when put together is a high risk factor for heart disease.

Basal Metabolism: The minimal amount of calories required to maintain life functions such as breathing and heartbeat.

Tropical Diet Taste Test©

Answer the following questions to determine your best Tropical Diet plan. When you get to the bottom of the list of questions, the column with the most circled yes answers will reveal the best plan for you to follow at this time.

If you want to skip the Taste Test, jump over to the program that suits your needs and calculate your daily calorie needs to determine your personal nutritional prescription.

Question	Tropical Diet Plan		
	Lean	*Athletic*	*Basic*
1. I do best on balanced nutritional programs			If yes
2. I lose weight fastest on high-protein diets.	If yes		
3. I am sugar-sensitive and crave carbohydrates.	If yes		
4. I do not exercise on a regular basis.	If yes		
5. I like to eat large portions of high-carb foods like fruits, vegetables, and grains.		If yes	
6. I like to have fat at every meal to help me feel full after meals.			If yes
7. I like to drink alcoholic beverages.			If yes
8. I like to eat meat, chicken, fish, and eggs on a regular basis.	If yes		
9. I am an active and athletic individual.		If yes	
10. I like to snack on chips, crackers, and fruit.		If yes	
11. I like to snack on protein-rich foods. like low-fat cheese, meat, nuts, and dairy	If yes		
12. I am a vegetarian.		If yes	
13. I like to eat small portions of food.	If yes		
14. I enjoy large volumes of food.		If yes	

My Tropical Diet Plan is: _____

After you determine your *L.A.B.* plan, it's time to do a little math. Don't let this scare you.

Just a little arithmetic will take you a long way. If you want some more math and science, you can always join the fitness-minded folks in the Athlete's section described in Chapter 6. In the meantime, the rest of you can take your ideal body weight, desirable body weight or your realistic weight goal and calculate your daily minimal calorie needs. This minimal amount of calories called the basal metabolic rate (BMR) is the amount of calories your body needs just to survive. The BMR is described in more detail in Chapter 6. For now, take your desired weight, multiply that weight by 10 calories per pound and viola! You have your calorie prescription in a jiffy.

Tropical Diet Calorie Formula

Take your desirable body weight x 10 calories per pound = daily calorie needs

---

Regardless of your test results, if you want to lose weight you will need to take out or work out 500-1,000 calories a day from *your normal* daily diet and exercise routine to lose at least ½ pound to 2.2 pounds per week. One way to calculate your normal dietary intake is by writing down a typical 24-hour dietary intake on the Tropical Diet Pocket Coach© chart. Add up the calories, carbohydrates, protein and fat in your foods by using the Tropical Diet Food Lists, or by referring to a food and calorie chart from most of the nutrition books listed in the references. Your Tropical Diet Nutritionist can also calculate your dietary intake using a computerized analysis program. All you need to do is log onto the website *www.thetropicaldiet.com.*

If your goal is to maintain your weight, to focus on sports performance to reduce blood fats, pressure, cholesterol or blood sugar reduction, then you'll need calculate your daily calorie intake based on your present weight. Add to that figure your total energy expenditure (TEE) and the specific dynamic action (SDA). These formulas and tables can be found in Chapter 6 in the *A*thlete's section.

In order to help you make your final decision about your *L.A.B.* plan and calorie prescription, I have included Tropical Dieter profiles, case studies of men and women I have counseled over the years. These profiles will help you to identify yourself in one of my ten clients who have converted their previous diet to my *L*ean, *A*thletic and *B*asic plans and have lost weight, changed their body shape, trained for their first marathon or Olympic qualifying event or dieted to lower cholesterol, blood sugars, or high blood pressure. Many of them tried unsuccessfully to lose weight on other programs. Here's how they learned to succeed.

Tropical Diet Profiles

Case One: *L*ean Plan. Switch to *A*thletic Plan for sports training when needed.

Lifestyle: Inconsistent eating schedule due to work and family responsibilities, social schedule, and premenopausal symptoms.

Goals: Feel more energetic, manage premenopausal symptoms, lose weight, and body fat gained recently.

Dietary recommendations: Healthier, more consistent food choices to manage sweet cravings and premenopausal symptoms.

Female
Age: 48
Height: 5'3"
Weight: 125 pounds

Dietary composition:	**Recommended *L*ean Plan:**
Calories: 1,400	Calories: 1,500 cal.
Carbohydrates: 97 g. (26%)	Carbohydrates: 189 g. (50%)
Protein: 76 g. (21%)	Protein: 52 to 72 g. (13-19 %)
Fat: 76 g. (47%)	Fat: 36 to 54 g. (21%-32%)

Morning

Coffee with milk
Honey Oats cereal with milk

Morning

½ c. soy based cereal with berries
soy milk, yogurt or soy fortified milk
fresh kiwi and/or citrus sections

Snack

Banana

Snack

apple with 1oz. fat-free jalapeno cheese

Afternoon

Chicken salad
Cole slaw
Cheddar cheese crackers
Diet soda

Afternoon

grilled chicken Caesar salad
with mandarin oranges, assorted
veggies, crushed toasted almonds
iced green tea

Snack

Chocolate chip cookie

Snack

EAS™ chocolate AdvantEdge® Drink or
½ PowerBar® sugar-free sport bar

Evening
2 glasses wine
salad with oil/vinegar
chicken marsala
cheesecake

Evening
1 glass red wine
spinach salad with carrots, tomatoes
and vinaigrette-oil free
grilled chicken breast with steamed
broccoli
fruit sorbet or frozen yogurt

Tropical Diet Profiles

Case Two: *A*thlete Plan

Lifestyle: Student athlete with hectic class and training schedule.

Goals: Lose weight and body fat, and feel more energetic for training and competition.

Dietary recommendations: high-carbohydrates, high-protein *A*thlete Plan

Female
Age: 28
Height: 5'8"
Weight: 160 pounds

Dietary composition:
Calories: 1,650
Carbohydrates: 226 g.
Protein: 60 g.
Fat: 56 g.

Recommended *A*thlete Plan:
Calories: 1,800 to 2,000
Carbohydrates: 250 to 325 g.
Protein: 80 to 100 g.
Fat: 44 to 66 g.

Breakfast
3 eggs sunny side up with
2 pieces of White toast
2 servings of Special K
with milk

Breakfast:
Egg white omelette with veggies
whole wheat toast, 1 tsp. soy butter
Special K cereal with raisins
and strawberries
1 c. skim, soy or fortified milk
1 cup fortified Tropicana® orange juice

Snack:
nothing

Snack
Clif LUNA™ Tropical Crisp bar

Afternoon
Fruit juice—Large

Afternoon
Fruit Smoothie with soy protein powder
or yogurt

Snack
nothing

Snack
TropCoco™coconut water or Propel
water with baked chips
and salsa

Dinner

Bowl of chili

Macaroni and cheese

Oreo cookies

Dinner

salad greens with carrots and

pasta with red sauce and parmesan

grilled vegetable assortment

Frozen yogurt—low fat, cookies and

cream flavor

Tropical Diet Profiles

Case Three: *B*asic Plan
Lifestyle: Lives life on the on the run with work, family responsibilities and a daily jog.
Goals: Improve food choices, eat healthier, feel better and get into better shape.
Dietary recommendations: First-time dieter to *B*asic Plan

Male
Age: 42
Height: 5'9"
Weight: 155 lbs.
Goal: Eat healthier, get into better shape, get more energetic

Dietary composition:
Calories: 1600
Carbohydrates: 178 g. (43%)
Protein: 99 g. (24%)
Fat: 59 g. (32%)

Recommended *B*asic Plan:
Calories: 1800
Carbohydrates: 194 g. (44%)
Protein: 120 g. (27%)
Fat: 56 g. (29%)

Early Morning after jog:
Nothing

Early Morning after jog:
water/ EAS™ AdvantEdge® Strawberry Drink

Morning
12 oz. water
5 oz. Apple Danish pastry
10 oz. water

Morning
water/ iced green tea
whole wheat bagel with 1 tsp. peanut butter and 1 tsp. apple butter
1 cup Tropicana® fortified O.J.

Snack
Nothing

Snack
apple with low-fat mozzarella stick

Afternoon
Turkey sandwich, white bread w/cheese, lettuce, tomato
3 oz. potato salad
1 dill pickle
1 peanut butter cookie
12 oz. Coca Cola

Afternoon
Turkey on whole wheat 6" sub with lettuce, tomato, pickle, green peppers mustard
1 low fat fruit yogurt
1 iced tea

Snack

Nothing

Dinner

Ham sandwich with mozzarella
cheese on potato bread
12 oz. water
1 bakery cookie

Snack

Genisoy® Extreme Island Blast Bar
or 1 oz. tropical trail mix
Water

Dinner

Lean meat sandwich on potato bread
with veggies, sprouts, mustard
12 oz. water
1 Tropical Brownie (see recipe
on page 217)

End-of-the-Chapter Questions

1. WHAT ARE THE PITFALLS OF FAD DIETS?

The experts at Tuft's University Health and Nutrition Center warn dieters against (see appendix for subscription information):

- Products and programs which promise quick fixes and results
- Any ad that says you can lose weight without paying attention to calories
- Any plan that eschews one or more of the food groups.

2. HOW DOES THE TROPICAL DIET COMPARE TO SUCCESS-FUL DIETERS WHO HAVE LOST 30 POUNDS OR MORE AND KEPT IT OFF FOR AT LEAST ONE YEAR AND RECORDED BY THE NATIONAL WEIGHT CONTROL REGISTRY?

- They lost weight through a combination of methods switching around to different plans as long as it worked, and is balanced.

The Tropical Diet offers you three plans, Lean, Athlete and Basic— and encourages you to try all the plans at some point during your dieting process.

- They have identified a weight loss trigger, special something that inspires them to lose weight.

The Tropical Diet helps you to identify your priority weight loss reasons and goals in Chapter 2 and by using the results from the Tropical Diet Taste Test.

- They have included daily exercise, averaging 4 miles of walking each day or the equivalent . . .

Exercise is encouraged from the first chapter. The exercise equivalents have been provided in the Athlete exercise section in Chapter 6.

- They do not make your diet all or nothing.

On the Tropical Diet, if you can't start a formal exercise program try something else like vacuuming the house, standing to work on the computer, or when watching TV instead of sitting. Even stretching in bed when you wake up will work. As for the diet, if you can't follow your L.A.B. plan five days a week, try it every other day or take the weekends off. Don't throw in your diet towel because you can't follow the program the whole 9 yards. By exercising or cutting just 200 calories worth each day, you can lose a minimum of 20 pounds this year alone!

• Monitor and measure your success.

The Tropical Diet helps you to keep track of your food intake and success with The Tropical Diet Pocket Coach© available with your book, through www.thetropicaldiet.com *website, or from your Tropical Diet Nutritionist.*

5

The Tropical ℒean Plan

Picture this. You've just been seated in the dining room of a luxurious resort overlooking the bright blue Caribbean sea, and your waiter offers you a sizzling cheese omelette dancing with a collage of green, red, and orange vegetables coupled with a papaya boat boasting an array of fresh pineapple, kiwi, guava, lychee, and grapes accompanied with a cup of strong island java and a freshly squeezed glass of orange juice.

This a just a taste of the ℒean Tropical Diet Plan menu you can prepare in the privacy of your own home.

In a nutshell, the Tropical Diet ℒean plan is a healthier version of many of the high-protein, low-carb diets that are popular today. The major difference between the other high-protein programs and the ℒean plan is that it is a scientifically and nutritionally modified version, which excludes the unhealthy aspects, retains the healthier features and fortifies the plan with essential carbohydrates—the minimal amount needed for long-term weight management, vital vitamins and minerals needed for energy, strength, and fiber—required for, well, let's just leave it at a smooth "passage."

The Tropical Diet ℒean program is for the protein-lover, the *Atkins*™ or *South Beach*© type- dieter or for those who feel better eating more protein instead of high-carbohydrates diets. We'll save the high-carbohydrate plan for the athletes and vegetarians. Don't get me wrong, however, vegetarians and athletes can also follow the ℒean plan if they give up some of their typical cereal, pasta, rice, or grain-based dishes in lieu of high-protein bars, or beverages, soy-based meals, and trail-mix snacks.

The ℒean program also caters to eaters who lose weight faster, and feel more energetic eating smaller portion sizes, and servings of grain, wheat, high-starch vegetables, fruits, and dairy.

While research shows that very-low carbohydrate diets such as Phase-1 *Atkins*™ and *South Beach*© can be risky to some dieters, there are actually some health benefits to low-carb plans, too. Low-carbohydrates diets may help accelerate the initial weight loss, to 2 to 13 pounds within the first week. And while this weight loss is often a result of water loss associated with eliminating carbohydrates, it feels good to lose weight quickly. Definitely a motivational boost at the onset of the diet program.

Probably the biggest difference between these other high-protein diets and the ℒean plan comes down to "the switch." Remember, by the 4th week of The Tropical Diet, you are actually encouraged to switch to one of the other *ℒ.𝒜.ℬ.* plans (see page 55) to boost your carbohydrate intake, replenish your body's carbohydrates stores (muscle and liver glycogen) and give your metabolism a kick. If you're really craving some carbs, you're encouraged to make the switch before that even happens

So, if your head over heels about high-protein diets, here's some additional validation that these programs work.

For example,

• There is a metabolic boost on high protein plans.
• A greater loss of heat in the form of calories (body temperature is slightly higher on a high-protein diet, therefore burning more calories over a day) occurs.
• A loss of calories in ketones found in urine, feces, and sweat (only on very low-carb diets of 50g or less)
• There is a preferential selection of nutrients moved towards building lean muscle mass and away from fat storage.

Additional benefits of the high-protein, low-carbohydrate plan may also include:

- Less hunger, better satiation after protein-rich meals, e.g., feeling more satisfied, fuller.
- Increased calorie burn when compared with high-carbohydrate diets.
- Higher diet-induced thermogenisis, more calories burned after the meal, about twice as much when compared with a high-carbohydrate diet, (especially after breakfast and dinner meals).
- Reduced blood triglyceride (fat) levels and cholesterol levels.
- Reduced overall hunger and suppressed appetite.
- Fewer calories consumed for dinner after high-protein lunches.
- Greater availability of food choices at restaurants and on the road, even at fast food restaurants like Wendy's, Burger King, and McDonald's.
- Lower blood sugar levels in late-onset diabetics.
- Access to hundreds of beverages, bars, and foods for _"convenience cuisine©"_ Tropical Dieters (see page 151).
- Syndrome Xers, those with metabolic syndrome or insulin resistance may do better on moderate carbohydrates (42 to 45%) and higher fat (35 to 40 %) diets than on high-carb diets excluding a weight loss and exercise program.

There are some drawbacks to high-protein, low-carbohydrate diets, too!

Over time, if you don't eat enough dietary carbohydrates, the body begins to burn stored carbohydrates for energy which releases a lot of water weight. The body also breaks down lean body tissue (muscle) in an effort to manufacture glucose (sugars) for energy and for the brain.

Here is some additional reasons why a very low-carbohydrate diet may be detrimental to some dieters' health.

1. Heart disease risk factors.
2. Increased cancer risk.
3. Poor long-term weight control.
4. Rising blood pressure with age.

5. Gout.
6. Kidney stones.
7. Osteoporosis.
8. Fainting.
9. Keto breath, which actually mimics alcohol breath which in addition to the dizziness and fainting on these diets may get you pulled over and arrested for DUI!

The Tropical Diet *Lean* program provides the lowest healthiest level of carbohydrates I am comfortable recommending, about 47 to 50% of the total calories (122 to 231 grams) on five caloric plans, from 1,000 to 2,000 calories. The nutritional composition for each *Lean* calorie level can be found in the Appendix. This minimal amount of carbohydrates will control cravings and keep you satisfied at mealtimes without enduring some of the unpleasant consequences associated with very-low-carbohydrate diets like ketosis, dizziness, headaches, nausea, and dehydration. It will keep the socially active person, professional homemaker, and volunteer energized and functioning for activities like household chores, carpools, childrearing, cocktail parties, and work. The program is not recommended for dieters who engage in serious sport training, daily exercise regimens, or strenuous activities like construction, landscaping, or professional childcare.

I have provided the profile of a *Lean* program candidate, a former follower of a popular high-protein, low-carbohydrate diet program who fell off the dietary wagon after a weekend on the carbohydrate town! He came to me to discuss ways to take his preferred high-protein dieting style by making it nutritionally balanced and long-lasting. This gentleman is a good example of the type of eater who would do best on this program. He shows you how The Tropical Diet can accommodate a high-protein diet while it improves the overall quality of his entire food and fluid intake. Here is an example of someone who may be just like you.

Male
Age: 36
Weight: 187
Height: 5'10"
Diet History: Followed a popular low-carb diet program and lost 13 pounds. Gained back 8 pounds.

Food Diary

Before	After

Before

Morning
1 scrambled egg
2 strips bacon
8 oz. 2% milk

After

Morning
½ c. scrambled Egg Beaters™ or egg white omelette
1 strip bacon
1 cup skim milk
½ cup mandarin orange sections

Snack
1 can diet soda

Snack
iced green tea
or 1 FUZE Tropical Slenderize Drink
1 oz. soy nuts

Afternoon
Chicken salad with
lettuce, tomato, peppers,
6 oz. turkey and mayo
1 can diet cola

Afternoon
6 oz. fresh turkey breast
lettuce, tomato, red pepper
onions and lite or lowfat salad
dressing
kiwi slices with mint

Snack
2 fried cheese sticks

Snack
2 oz. lowfat string cheese
1 apple

Evening
Chicken Caesar salad
16 oz. steak

Evening
Tossed dark green or spinach salad
w/carrots, tomato, onion, peppers
6 oz. salmon
½ cup peas
1 cup steamed broccoli
½ cup sliced papaya

Snack
2 sugar-free popsicles

1 liter water
throughout the day

Snack
same snack

bottled water with lemon, orange or
key lime slices

Lean Program Menu and Snack Choices

On the _Lean_ program, the best way to think of your daily meal choices is to imagine a handful of protein-rich foods, about 4 to 6 oz. at each meal—eggs, fish, non-fat cheese, chicken, turkey, lean meats, and pork, served with generous portions of colorful vegetables, a few slices of tropical fruit, and pinch of fat from oil, nuts, or additional fats contributed from the cooking process.

Your personal plan looks like this:

Calories	1000	1200	1500	1800	2100
Food Groups:					
Milk	1 cup	2 cups	2 cups	3 cups	3 cups
Fruit	4 fruits	5 fruits	6 fruits	6 fruits	7 fruits
Vegetables	2 cups	3 cups	3 cups	3 cups	3 cups
Grains	2	2	3	4	4
Protein	8 oz.	10 oz.	12 oz.	13 oz.	15 oz.
Fat	3 tsp.	3 tsp.	3 tsp.	4 tsp.	6 tsp.

The *Lean* Guide to Meals

Here is your guide to meal planning. The key to eating the *Lean* style diet is to emphasize protein based foods at all meals and snacks, seasoned with vegetables, fruits, fluids, and a small amount of grains and fats. Additional *Lean* menu choices can be found in Chapter 8.

Meals	Food Servings	Examples
Breakfast	2 protein servings or 1 dairy	egg white omelette or fat free yogurt
	1 fruit	orange or berries
Snack	1 protein or 1 fat 1 oz. soy nuts	1 low fat string cheese
Lunch	3 to 4 protein 1 to 2 cups vegetables 1 fat	4 oz. grilled chicken breast on green vegetable salad 1 tbsp. low fat dressing
Snack	2 fruits	berry smoothie with protein
	1 protein	powder supplement scoop or apple slices with lowfat cheese
Dinner	1 cup vegetables 3 to 4 protein 2 starch	1 cup vegetable soup 3-4 oz. grilled fish 1 cup potatoes or yellow rice
	1 fat	1 tsp. butter for potato or oil used in rice preparation

The best way to add a tropical twist is to garnish the dishes with tropical fruits, fresh steamed vegetables, or to season your dish with a dab of Tabasco sauce, hot sauce, ginger, curry, or fresh herbs like mint, parsley, basil, or cilantro.

A Day in the Life of the Lean Plan

Wake-up call
Iced tea or coffee with fat-free ½ and ½

Bottled water

Rationale:
caffeine speeds up the metabolism

important on high-protein diets

Breakfast
Egg white omelette with veggies
½ c. tropical fruit cup with grapefruit

alternative:
EAS™ AdvantEdge® drink
or
low-carb cereal with berries

Mid-morning snack
LifeLine nonfat cheese with
apple slices

soy nuts

Lunch
1 turkey or chicken salad with veggies
lettuce, tomato, cucumber,
green peppers, and mustard
Iced tea with lemon

clear vegetable consume
grilled fish with vegetables

Afternoon Snack
Ginger tea with lemon

frozen fruit pop

Evening
Green salad with carrots, tomatoes,
onions and fat-free dressing
grilled chicken breast
with steamed green veggies

jicama sticks with salsa
Pam-fried Cuban steak
with fruit chutney

Snack
Sugar-free frozen yogurt cone

frozen blueberries with lowfat
whipped cream

End-of-the-Chapter Questions

1. WHAT ARE SOME OF THE DRAWBACKS TO THE HIGH-PROTEIN, LOW-CARBOHYDRATE POPULAR DIET PROGRAMS?

They:

- Are too low in carbohydrates for active individuals, as in the level found in *The Zone Diet* (25 to 40%), *Atkins*™ (5 to 18%), *Sugar Busters*™ (40%) and *Protein Power*™ (8 to 14%).
- Could lead to excessive fat, saturated fat, and cholesterol intake if low-fat, lean protein foods are not selected.
- Could be costly depending on the quality and amount of daily protein and protein supplements consumed.
- May affect the kidney, resulting in elevated blood urea nitrogen (BUN) levels if carbohydrates are limited to 25% of total calories.
- May lead to the buildup of nitrogen, in which it needs to be cleaned from the blood and gotten rid of as urea in urine. This nitrogen-urea effect can cause dehydration, further straining the kidneys. Kidney care is crucial since there is no cure for kidney failure.
- May set up the body for kidney stones.
- Require extra time-consuming attention for the selection and preparation of low-fat, low-cholesterol, and low saturated fat sources for long-term health lipid profiles.

2. HOW IS THE TROPICAL DIET LEAN PROGRAM DIFFERENT FROM POPULAR HIGH-PROTEIN, LOW-CARB DIET PROGRAMS?

The Tropical Diet provides a healthier ratio of carbohydrates, protein, and fat and ensures an adequate vitamin and mineral intake and fiber for healthy bathroom experiences.

3. WHAT IF I CRAVE CARBOHYDRATES ON THIS PLAN?

Then make the switch . . . try another Tropical Diet *L.A.B.* plan for a day or a week to replenish glycogen stores (see page 55).

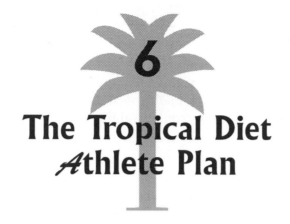

The Tropical Diet
*A*thlete Plan

This chapter strikes a personal chord in my heart since this is the place where my personality, professional accomplishments, and soul resides.

I was born an athlete, grew up participating in almost every competitive sport, and matured into a professional triathlete in my 30s. Today at 43 years young, I remain highly competitive in running, and multisport, having competed in hundreds of road, cross-country, trail, and endurance races, triathlons including the Ironman in Lake Placid, New York, and 31 marathons, coming just a few minutes off of qualifying for the US Marathon Olympic Trials in 1996. My personal best running times are approximately 17 minutes for the 5K, 37 minutes for the 10 K, 1:20 for the half marathon, and 2:52 for the full marathon. My best times were recorded at the Boston (2:53), Los Angeles (2:53), and Walt Disney World (2:52) marathons. In addition, I have won scores of races nationwide. Recently, I qualified for the World Long Distance Duathlon Championships, representing the United States on Team USA in Denmark, 2004.

I believe my tropically nutritious diet has contributed 99.9% to the success of my races, recovery from training, and competition and prevention of injuries in over 20 years of competition. And, it has been a tasty adventure, too!

Here's how the *A*thlete plan can help you.

The Tropical Diet *A*thlete plan is designed for the fitness-minded, athletic individual. Whether you're training for your favorite sport or interested in losing body fat and weight while engaging in regular physical activity, this program is for you. It is also an ideal program for vegetarians.

The *A*thlete plan is a high-complex-carbohydrate, low-fat program with five calorie levels from 1,200 to 2,400 calories. It provides a minimum of 55% carbohydrates and less than 20% fat to enhance glycogen storage in muscles and limit excessive dietary fat. The nutritional composition of the *A*thlete plan can be found on page 268.

The advantages of the *A*thlete plan for sport includes:

- All sports including anaerobic ones like dancing, skating, and tennis, and aerobic sports like running, swimming, and cycling rely on the availability of carbohydrate fuel.
- Simple and complex carbohydrates contribute to the primary fuel needed for sport.
- A carbohydrate intake of approximately 50 to 75% total calories has been recommended for sport training.
- Approximately 4 grams carbohydrates/kg bodyweight for 1 to 2 hours of daily training is the minimal amount advised to maintain adequate glycogen stores for long distance training. Up to 8 to 10 grams carbohydrate/kg BW may be required for intense daily training of more than 2 to 4 hours daily (over 70% maximum heart rate which is 220 minus your age).
- Carbohydrate-rich diets (65% or higher) enhance the immune system during training when compared with low-carbohydrate, high-fat diets.

For weight loss:

- Participants in the National Weight Control Registry who include 3000+ registrants who have kept the weight off for more than 6 years contribute their success in part by eating a low-fat, high-carbohydrate diet.
- High-carbohydrate, high-fiber meals help fill up dieters, a weight

control aid especially when the high-fiber, carbohydrate foods are eaten at breakfast.

High-carbohydrate, low-fat diets have also recently been given the thumbs-up by popular diet book authors. Despite all the negative carbo-publicity and dieters-obsession with carbohydrate avoidance, high-carbohydrate diets have repeatedly been shown to help individuals lose weight.

A meta-analysis, a comprehensive look at many dietary studies on high-carb diets, has demonstrated an average weight loss of 22 pounds in individuals who started with an initial higher body weight. In addition, the United States Dept. of Agriculture (USDA) recently released a study on 10,014 adults across the U.S. which showed that high-carb dieters consume 300 fewer calories day and were more likely to be in the normal weight range than very low-carb dieters.

There are four main reasons why high carbohydrate, low-fat diets are preferred over high-fat diets to limit excessive weight gain:

- Dietary fat above energy requirements is stored in adipose tissue and does not stimulate fat oxidation.
- High-fat diets have a weak satiating effect and promote a passive overconsumption of calories.
- Low-fat diets followed for a period of 2 months or more provide a significant weight loss difference of 7 pounds more than high fat diets and may be more beneficial in maintaining weight loss.
- Low-fat diets are advocated to lower the risk of coronary heart disease and certain forms of cancer.

Popular diet programs such as *Atkins*™ (50 to 80% fat), the *Zone*™ (30 to 55% fat) *Sugar Busters*™ (40% or more fat), and *Protein Power*™ (66 to 83% fat) provide beyond reasonable and healthy dosages of fat for most athletic individuals.

And for health:

- More compatible with healthy eating guidelines than popular low-carbohydrate diet programs.
- The high-carbohydrate nations of Asia including China (less than

15%), Republic of Korea (22%), Thailand (20%) and Japan (3%) all have extremely low rates of obesity when compared with the U.S.

- A USDA study among others showed that high-carbohydrate diets provide more vitamins A, C, carotene and folate, the minerals calcium, magnesium, and iron than low-carbohydrate diets.
- Less than 20% fat, also ideal for cholesterol reduction.
- Phytochemical rich diet for overall health and longevity.
- France's and Italy's diet which consists of more bread and pasta than Americans have a much lower incidence of obesity 31% and 37%, respectively, when compared with the U.S. (61%).

The disadvantages are:

- High-carbohydrate diets loaded with high glycemic index foods greater than 70 (see end-of-the-chapter questions) can result in insulin resistance, your body's way of having difficulty keeping your blood sugars within normal range. However, this effect can be modulated by activity—many of the Tropical Diet foods, fruits, and vegetables do not exceed this limit.

- May be too high in carbohydrates and simple carbs for sugar-sensitive and carbohydrate-craving dieters.
- May cause water retention.
- More difficult to control portion size.
- May cause a laxative effect in some who are not accustomed to eating large portions of vegetables, fruits, and grains.

Athlete Energetics

Probably the major difference between the *A*thlete plan and the *L*ean and *B*asic program other than the greater carbohydrate allowance are the additional mathematical calculations recommended for accurate calorie, carbohydrate, fat, and protein needs.

Now, by no means do you have get out the calculator and start figuring out your requirements. In fact, you can take the simple equation of calculating daily calorie needs outlined in Chapter 4 and add your daily exercise and SDA calories to figure out your total energy needs. However, my recommendation is to get a more accurate picture to help maintain your weight, muscle mass, and health so you can train day-after-day without injury, illness or weight loss. Here are just some of the areas you need to know best.

Daily Calorie Needs

As you recall from Chapter 4 there are three factors which impact your calorie needs, the basal metabolic rate (BMR), the calories expended for physical activity, and the calories expended for the digestion of food, otherwise known as the SDA. For the basal calories, you can use the simple formula of desirable weight x 10 calories per pound to get your BMR or you can use one of the following formulas which are gender and/or age dependent.

Formulas for Calculating Daily Energy Needs

Formula One:

Men	Women
1 calorie/kg body weight/hour	.9 cal/kg/hour

Use this formula to calculate kilogram (kg) body weight =
Weight in pounds/2.2

If you want to weigh 125 pounds (57 kg) and you are:

Male*, take 1 calorie/57 kg/24 hours	=1,368 calories
Female, .9 calories/57 kg/24 hours	=1,231 calories

---

*I realize most men do not want to weigh that low amount, however I chose to go with the same weight to demonstrate the difference your gender makes on your calorie needs.

This other formula I frequently use with more competitive athletes is neither age nor gender dependent, but is dependent on lean body mass, your weight minus your percentage body fat. It's called the Cunningham Formula and is described in my last book, _The_

Vegetarian Sports Nutrition Guide (Wiley, 2000). For using this formula, you will need to know your percentage body fat. It provides a more accurate caloric picture of BEE for the more active person.

Cunningham Formula

Calculating Basal Energy Expenditure for Active Individuals

You'll need to know your percentage body fat to use this formula

Basal Energy Expenditure (BEE) = 500+ 22 (Fat Free Mass)•

———————

*Body weight in kg; FFM in kg
** (FFM) Fat Free Mass (kg) = Total kg weight—% body fat in kg

Example: 24 year-old, 125 pound (57kg) female with 12% body fat.
BEE = 500 + 22 (57- 6.84 (57 x .12) =
500 + (22 x 50.1) =
500 + 1103.5 = 1,603.5 calories

Exercise Calories

The energy expended for activity is the most variable component of your total calorie needs. It may range from 10% of total calorie needs if you're a couch potato to 50% of total needs in the competitive athlete. The energy expended for physical activity (EEPA) depends on:

• Body size.
• Efficiency of individual habits.
• Variations in body mass.

Excess postexercise oxygen consumption (EPOC) also affects energy expenditure. EPOC is the amount of calories you burn even after your exercise session. This can account for an additional 8 to 14% increase in your metabolic rate so it's worth it if you're trying to lose weight, have hit a plateau, or just want to eat more food every day.

Don't wait!

You better get started on your exercise plan, because like the BMR, calories expended for exercise (EEPA) declines with age. This is probably because of the natural tendency for body fat to increase and muscle mass to decline as you age.

For simplicity sake, the easiest way to calculate calories expended for exercise is to use the five-level classification of physical work, which I adapted from several exercise physiology textbooks. More detailed charts on specific activities can be found in most college sports science textbooks.

The categories listed in the table below provide calories expended for very light to exhausting physical work. In order to calculate your exercise calorie expenditure you need to write down all your daily activities, multiply the time you spend in the activity by the amount of approximate calories listed in the chart and total all the numbers to get your daily calorie expenditure.

Based on my hands-on experience, it is best to go with the most conservative amount of calories expended. You can always add more calories if you are losing too much weight, or if you want to maintain or gain weight.

Table 3
Classification of Activities Based on Intensity

Activity Level	Activity	Calories used Male	Female
Very light	sleeping, lying, reading, driving, ironing, sewing, watching TV, dish-washing, carpentry, painting, typing, laundry	1-1.5 calories per minute for both sexes	
Light	walking 2.5–3.5 mph, shopping, bowling, golf, pleasure sailing, table tennis, fishing, sweeping the floor	2-4.9 cal/min	1.5-3.4 cal/min
Moderate	pleasure cycling, dancing, volleyball, dancing, badminton and calisthenics-stretching/pilates, scrubbing floors, weeding, hoeing, tennis	5-7.4 cal/min	2.8-5.3 cal/min

Activity Level	Activity	Calories used	
		Male	**Female**
Heavy	ice skating, water skiing, competitive tennis, jogging, novice mountain climbing, pick and shovel work, walking uphill with load, swimming, boxing	7.5-9.9 cal/min	4.4-5.9 cal/min
Very Heavy	fencing, touch football, scuba diving, basketball, swimming, climbing, rowing	10-12.4 cal/min	6-7.5 cal/min
Unduly Heavy	handball, squash, cross-country skiing, running fast, hard cycling	12.5 & up cal/min	9.5 & up cal/min

---

Sample Chart for Calculating
Daily Calorie Expenditure for Activities and Exercise

A typical energy expending day in the life of the 125 pound (57 kg) 12% fat school crossing guard:

Activity	time	calories expended	
Sleeping, sitting, driving	8 hours	1 x 60 min x 8 hours =	480 calories
Standing/walking	4 hours	1.3 x 60 x 4 hours =	312 calories
Golf	1 hour	2.4 x 60 =	144 calories

Total estimated calories used for activity: 936 calories

Total Calories for BEE & exercise (125 pounds) = (1603.5 + 936) 2,539 calories

Calories for Food Metabolism

The total expenditure for food (TEF) or specific dynamic action (SDA) calories, the amount of calories you use to digest, absorb, metabolize, and synthesize protein, carbohydrates, and fats varies with the composition of your diet. However, it is estimated to be 10% of the basal metabolic rate (BMR) plus the energy expended for physical activity (EEPA.) While the jury is still out, research has shown the things you can do to boost or use more calories in this department. These ways are listed on page 55.

To calculate the number expended for SDA calories using the 125-pound individual example from above, BMR + EEPE calories = 2,539

SDA calories = 2539 x .10 = 253 calories

Total Daily Calorie Needs

The total daily calorie needs for the sample individual is:
2,539 + 253 calories = 2,792 calories

The Tropical Diet Plan for this person to lose weight safely can range from 1,500 calories (BMR calorie estimate)—1800 calories. This person can increase the amount of calories if she or he includes regular exercise and if he or she continues to lose 1 to 2 pounds a week.

You can calculate your weight maintenance plan by calculating the BEE, EEPA and SDA after you reach their desirable weight. The maintenance calories may be as high as 2,100 to 2,600 calories.

Tropical Diet Energetics: Calculating Energy Needs

1. Take your BMR:
Basal energy needs (BMR) the minimum amount of energy required to maintain the metabolic needs for basic body functions such as blood circulation, breathing, kidney function, and constant body temperature. You can calculate this number by using the formulas on page 89 & 90. The simplest method to use is to take your desirable weight and multiply it by 10 calories per pound.

2. Add your BMR to Daily Activities:
Calculate your daily energy expenditure from daily activities using the charts on pages 91–92. You can either add up each individual activity or you can use the simpler conversion ballpark factors listed on page 53.

3. Take the sum of your BMR and daily activity calories and multiply that number by 10% (.10) for the SDA.

Your total Daily Energy Expenditure can be calculated this way:

BMR calories + Daily activity calories + [(BMR calories + daily activity calorie) x 10%] = the amount of calories it takes to digest, metabolize, and assimilate the food you consume.

TEF Calorie-Burning Boosters

There are actually ways you can boost the calories you use in this department. These tips are especially useful if you're the vegetarian dieter or high-carb dieter looking to lose weight

- Eat high-carbohydrate meals and high-protein meals instead of fat.
- Eat protein-rich meals, especially at breakfast and dinner.
- Add spicy foods like red pepper and chilies to your meals. Spicy foods also enhance and prolong the effect of TEF. Meals with chili and mustard may increase the metabolism as much as 33% when compared with unspiced meals, and this effect may last for more than 3 hours.
- Drink beverages with caffeine if your health permits it. One cup of coffee (100 mg) consumed every two hours can increase the TEF by 8 to 11%. Nicotine will also stimulate the TEF, however smoking is not a healthy weight control method. It does explain why smokers might gain weight after giving up the habit. The best thing a smoker can do is give it up and start to exercise, which will counteract this effect.

A Day in the Life of the Athlete Plan

Wake-up call
Iced tea or coffee with fat-free half & half
Propel water

Rationale:
caffeine spares muscle glycogen
fluids prevent dehydration

Before Workout
Gatorade® or Accelerade®

Training carbohydrate needs:
take ½ body weight in pounds and drink/eat in carbohydrate grams.

During training session
Gatorade® or Accelerade®, Power gel®,
GU® or Jog mate®

25-30 grams of carbs per half hour
to prevent low blood sugar, or glycogen depletion. Can be beverage, sport bar, or gel.

Within 30 minutes of training
EAS™ AdvantEdge® drink or
sugar-free Power Bar®

1.5 grams carbohydrates per
kilogram body weight to replenish
glycogen stores. 1.5 grams per kg
bodyweight every two hours after.
High glycemic index foods best.
May also benefit from 4:1 ratio
carbs to protein for muscle recovery
and repair.

*A*thlete Plan Menu and Snack Choices

On the *A*thlete plan, you will find all the same foods and menu
suggestions as the *L*ean food plan however, additional portions of
carbohydrate-based foods like pastas, rice, couscous, potatoes, and
grains are also included. Visualize your plate with a handful of
chicken, fish, or meat with fruits, vegetables, and sport drinks, sport
bars, gels, and beverages to fuel the active Tropical Dieter.

Your personal plan looks like this:

Calories	1200	1500	1800	2000	2400
Food Groups:					
Milk	2 cups	2 cups	3 cups	3 cups	3 cups
Fruit	6 fruits	7 fruits	8 fruits	8 fruits	8 fruits
Vegetables	3 cups	3 cups	3 cups	3 cups	3 cups
Grains	3	4	5	6	9
Protein	5 oz.	6 oz.	8 oz.	10 oz.	12 oz.
Fat	2 tsp.	3 tsp.	4 tsp.	4 tsp.	6 tsp.

The Athlete Guide to Meals

Here is your guide to meal planning. The key to eating the Athlete style diet is to emphasize carbohydrate-based foods at all meals and snacks, seasoned with protein, vegetables, fruits, fluids, and a small amount of fats. Additional Athlete menu choices can be found in Chapter 8.

Meals	Food Servings	Examples
Breakfast	2 protein servings or 1 dairy	egg white omelette or fat-free yogurt
	1 to 2 starches	2 slices toast
	1 fruit	orange or berries
Snack	1 protein or 1 fat	1 low-fat string cheese or 1 oz. soy nuts, 1 apple
	1 fruit	or trail mix
Lunch	3 to 4 protein	4 oz. grilled chicken breast
	1 to 2 cups vegetables	on green vegetable salad
	1 fat	1 tbsp. low-fat dressing
	1 to 2 starch	2 sourdough rolls
Snack	2 fruits	berry smoothie with protein
	1 protein	powder supplement scoop
		or
		apple slices with low-fat cheese
	1 starch	whole grain pretzels
	or	
	sport bar/beverage	
Dinner	1 cup vegetables	1 cup vegetable soup
	3 to 4 protein	3-4 oz. grilled fish
	2 starch	1 cup potatoes or yellow rice
	1 fat	1 tsp. butter for potato or oil used in rice preparation

Typical Meal Plan

Breakfast
egg white omelette with veggies
fresh tropical fruit cup
1 slice 7-grain toast with low-sugar jam
Café con leche

For vegetarians:
egg substitute
soy sports beverage or smoothie
soy cheese with toast/apple
coffee with soy milk

Mid-morning snack
1 Tropical Crisp LUNA™ bar

Low sugar
PowerBar® Protein Plus™-sugar free

Lunch
1 turkey or chicken sub with veggies
lettuce, tomato, cucumber, green peppers,
and mustard on whole wheat bread
1 bag baked chips
1 apple
Ice tea with lemon

Vegetarian
veggie sub with low-fat cheese,
baked chips
fruit salad
yogurt

Afternoon Snack

Berry smoothie with added soy protein

fresh apple with Genisoy Tropical
paradise Trail Mix

Evening
green salad with carrots, tomatoes, onions,
fat-free dressing
2 whole-grain rolls with Benecol spread
6 oz. grilled chicken breast
with steamed green veggies
frozen non-fat or lowfat yogurt cone
FUZE beverage, Syfo or Arizona
sparkling water

same

same
grilled veggie
burger
same

Snack
air-blown popcorn with parmesan cheese
or
frozen yogurt with fresh fruit topping

No calories/low-sugar
Heavenly Desserts™ Meringue

frozen unsweetened yogurt cone

End-of-the-Chapter Questions

1. WHAT IS THE GLYCEMIC INDEX (GI). HOW CAN I USE THE GI NUMBERS FOR WEIGHT CONTROL, PEAK PERFORMANCE, AND LIFE?

In healthy people, the pancreas secretes enough insulin to move excess blood sugar from the bloodstream into the body's cells. When you have high blood sugar, your pancreas produces too little insulin to handle a sugar load. Therefore, it was assumed that anyone with high blood sugars or sugar sensitivities would benefit from eating complex carbohydrates since their fiber and complex sugar molecules content gives the pancreas a heads up and time to produce enough insulin to curb the sugar peak.

That all changed about 24 years ago when a group of researchers from the Jenkin's group put hundreds of foods to the test and measured the effect of the individual food on the blood sugar response during the first 2 hours of consumption and compared it to the response of pure sugar which scores a 100 on the scale. This scale, called the glycemic index (GI), is a widely recognized classification tool ranking foods according to their GI effect.

In 1997, the Food and Agriculture Association (FAO) and the World Health Organization (WHO) reviewed all the data regarding carbohydrates and health and determined that the GI index was a reliable method for classifying carbohydrate foods which can be used in conjunction with information about food composition to guide food choices. The committee recommends the consumption of a 55% carbohydrate diet with the bulk coming from low GI index foods.

The tool has been accepted with caution. The American Dietetic Association and the American Diabetes Association do not endorse the glycemic index as a weight loss program. The American Diabetes Association has pointed out that the first priority should be given to the total amount of carbohydrate instead of the source of carbohydrate.

And recently, experts have noted that many healthful foods have higher glycemic indexes than less nutritionally desirable foods. For example, carrots score very high, and whole milk ice cream scores very low. They do not see a consensus for supporting the glycemic index as a diet plan because:

- Glycemic index food tables are inconsistent.
- Combined foods have a different rank from single foods.
- Different combinations of foods have not been analyzed for glycemic index, therefore, it is not a practical tool for everyday life.

The key to using the GI index to your best interest is to make the healthiest food choices in general and use the index as one more way to choose between one food over another from the same food group. For instance, oatmeal (65) may be a better choice than a bagel (72) for breakfast, while an apple (36) could be a better fruit snack instead of watermelon (72). Choosing low glycemic index foods exclusively may not assist in your weight loss, sport performance, or total health since many of the low GI foods are loaded with fat such as whole milk (27), M&Ms (33), and sponge cake (46). We know this type of diet over the long run can increase the risk of heart disease, cancer, stroke, and obesity. Portion-controlling high GI foods like shredded wheat (69), whole wheat bread (69), and cantaloupe (65) may be more nutritious in the long run.

Tropical Diet suggestions for benefitting from the selection of low GI snacks and meals:
- Select the lower GI—geared Tropical Diet Plans, *L*ean and *B*asic if you are sugar-sensitive.
- If you choose the *A*thlete plan for sport training select low GI starches, fruits, and vegetables for main meals and snacks.
- Select low-carb drinks, bars, and foods designed for diabetics or athletes listed in Tropical Diet Foundation Food List on page 128–130 such as the Bristol-Meyers Squib Choice Bars, sugar-free PowerBars and EAS™ and Accelerade drinks.
- Select trail mix, tomato soup, yogurt, fruit smoothies prepared with soy or yogurt for in-between meals.
- Choose low-GI fruits such as strawberries, frozen grapes, or a few dried apricots.
- Have a bowl of oatmeal with raisins and cinnamon.
- Have an apple a day to keep. Well, you know the rest!

Glycemic Index of Tropical Diet Foods

VERY LOW Under 39	LOW 40-54	MODERATE 55-69	HIGH equal or Greater than 70
smoothie with soy	orange juice	figs	Gatorade™
protein	pineapple juice	raisins	Kavli™ Crackers
skim milk	grapes	condensed milk	pancakes
pear	low-fat ice cream	bran chex	Cheerios™
peach	All Bran™	Grape nuts™	corn flakes
apple	special K	muesli	puffed wheat
fresh &	old-fashioned oats	quick oats	bagel
dried apricots	brown rice	honey	pretzels
cherries	oat bran bread	shredded wheat	white bread
grapefruit	pumpernickel	Ryvita™ crackers	carrots
plum	rye bread	pita bread	instant potatoes
prickly pear	apple muffin	sourdough bread	watermelon
strawberries	corn tortilla	pizza	rice cakes
sugar-free fruit	taro	bran muffin	melba toast
yogurt	parsnips	stone ground whole	white rice
fruit yogurt	sweet potato	wheat bread	saltines
with sugar	green peas	whole wheat bread	water crackers
lima beans	banana	angel food cake	graham cracker
barley	orange	beets	vanilla wafers
egg fettuccine	kiwi	corn	Clif™ Bar
whole wheat spaghetti	black beans	potato	MetRx™ Bar
chickpeas	black eyed peas	mango	jelly beans
kidney beans	apple juice	papaya	Life Savers™
lentils	banana bread	pineapple	
Ironman™ sport bar	cassava	udon noodles	
navy beans	raisins	popcorn	
soybeans	soba noodles	couscous	
split peas & soup	cornmeal	wild rice	
chocolate		PowerBar®	
tomato soup			
peanuts, M&Ms™			
fructose			

2. How do vitamins and minerals give me energy?

Vitamins and minerals do not give energy. However, they are the links and regulators of energy-producing and muscle-building pathways. There are two different groups of vitamins, the water-soluble and the fat-soluble. This property determines how they are absorbed, transported, excreted, and stored in the body.

Water-soluble Vitamins B and C

B-vitamins include thiamin (B1), riboflavin (B2), niacin (B3), pyridoxine (B6), cobalamin (B12), folic acid, pantothenic acid, and biotin work in every cell. These Bs make it possible for the body to use carbohydrates, proteins, and fats for fuel that makes them essential for energy use. Some B-vitamin needs increase pro-portionally with calorie expenditure.

That means if you're more active, you need to eat more vitamin B-rich food and beverages. That's easy to do on The Tropical Diet, especially since the foods that happen to begin with the letter B are brown like beef, pork, whole grains, beans, and legumes. Fortified beverages like Propel water, cereals, sport bars, and even Tropicana orange juice also have B-vitamins.

As for vitamin C, it also helps you to metabolize the calories from food, so you need to get enough vitamin C to feel energized too! Fortunately almost all of the tropical fruits and vegetables contain vitamin C so it's not hard to find on this program.

Fat-soluble Vitamins

Fat-soluble vitamins A, D, E, and K are stored in the liver and fat deposits of your body. Your body can survive weeks without consuming fat-soluble vitamin-rich foods, as long as you get them in the long run. Many Tropical Diet food choices have the essential fat-soluble vitamins.

Here's a handy chart you can use to track down the vitamins in your diet to make sure you get enough on a regular basis.

Water-soluble Vitamins and Food Sources

B¹ Thiamin
pork, seeds, black beans, green peas, watermelon, oatmeal, baked potato

B² Riboflavin
milk, spinach, mushrooms, enriched grains
and soy products, green papaya

B³ Niacin
tuna, chicken, enriched grains, peanuts,beef,
mushrooms, baked potato

B⁶ Pyridoxine
baked potato, watermelon, banana, meat,
spinach, navy beans, broccoli, sweet potato,
avocado

B¹² Cobalamin
fortified products—cereals, breads, animal
products

Folic Acid
spinach, turnip greens, lima beans,
beets, asparagus, broccoli, OJ, winter
squash, cantaloupe, organ meats, blood
and navel oranges, artichokes

Pantothenic acid
whole grains, legumes, meat

Biotin
synthesized in gut, liver, egg yolks

Vitamin C
orange juice, broccoli, cantaloupe, brussel
sprouts, green pepper, tomatoes and
juice, baked potato, artichokes, cranberries,
kale, kiwi, blood and navel oranges,
persimmons, pomegranates, cabbage, bok
choy, artichokes, chestnuts, sweet potatoes,
green papaya, lotus root

Fat-Soluble Vitamins and Food Sources

Vitamin A
carrots, greens, sweet potato, butternut
squash, cantaloupe fortified "milks," liver,
green papaya, persimmons, sweet potato

Vitamin D
natural sunlight; fortified margarine, milks,
egg yolk, liver, fish, tuna, salmon

Vitamin E
vegetable oils, leafy greens, nuts, seeds, sweet
potato, wheat germ

Vitamin K
synthesized in intestinal tract, beef, liver, cabbage type vegetables, leafy greens

Minerals

Minerals are natural compounds that your body needs for enzyme and chemical reaction facilitation within the body. Here is a quick look at the minerals and food sources from your Tropical Diet foods. If you are interested in learning more about vitamins and minerals, several nutrition books listed in Appendix A are excellent resources.

Mineral Tropical Food Sources

Calcium
dairy products, tofu, greens, legumes, green papaya, sea vegetables, buckwheat, broccoli, bok choy, bony fish

Phosphorus
cereals and baked goods, meat, dairy

Magnesium
nuts, legumes, whole grains, dark greens, chocolate and cocoa

Sodium
table salt, sea salt, soy sauce, soups, frozen foods, cheese, processed foods like crackers, chips, cookies, cold cuts

Chloride
table salt, soy sauce

Potassium
fruits, vegetables, grains, legumes, cranberries, artichokes, oranges, kiwi, sweet potato, cabbage

Sulfur
all protein-containing foods, preservatives

Iron
whole or enriched grains, dried fruits, legumes, leafy greens, tofu fermented miso, soy sauce, liver, roast beef, green papaya

Iodine
iodized salt, plants grown in iodized soil

Zinc
nuts, seeds, whole grains, tofu and beef, pork, chicken thigh, yogurt

Copper
nuts, seeds, artichokes, sweet potato

Fluoride
tea, toothpaste

Selenium
grains and vegetables dependent on soil conditions, eggs, seafood, and organ meats, steak

Chromium
grains, nuts, and organ meats

Molybdenum
grains, legumes, and organ meats

Manganese
nuts, whole grains

Cobalt
whole wheat, bran, B12

3. DO YOU NEED TO TAKE A VITAMIN/MINERAL SUPPLE-MENT WHILE FOLLOWING THE TROPICAL DIET?

Fortunately if you follow your *L.A.B.* plan and menus, you are likely to eat a variety of tropical foods including meats, chicken, vegetables, fruits, grains, and dairy and therefore will get most of the vitamins and minerals you need on a daily basis. However, it is impossible to control the vitamin content of all foods or control your daily eating habits or other factors such as medication needs, activity patterns, food preparation techniques, all of which affect the vitamin and mineral content of foods.

What supplement(s) should you take?

At some point in life, you may need to consider supplementation.

Why? Because you're not perfect, you do not live in a perfect world, and thus because your life changes from day-to-day, so do your dietary needs.

Just imagine, if you don't get to the grocery this week and run out of meats, fruits, veggies, milk, or cereal, you might be at risk at missing out on an entire food group! That's where the dietary supplement steps in. Other opportunities for supplementation include childhood and adolescence, pregnancy and lactation, trauma and emotional stress (look for my next book on this topic) and, of course, sports training, competition, and recovery.

Now don't get me wrong. I really prefer you get your vitamins and minerals through food but you may have unusual circumstances or needs which require you to get a daily dose from somewhere else. And it doesn't necessarily mean from a pill. Supplements come in all forms—shakes, drinks, bars, and powders.

And, while I have my own favorite list of favorite supplements, there are thousands more on the market and new ones as we speak. The ones I have listed here are based on taste, effectiveness, product quality, availability, and client acceptability from youngsters to seniors, recreational exercisers to Olympian athletes.

And while supplements and their manufacturers may have updated formulas from time to time, I can only give you the most recent update I have at the publishing of this book. Remember that not all supplements are safe for everyone all the time, so please check with your physician, or registered dietitian (RD) before consuming any new food, supplement, or beverage unfamiliar to you.

Don't be surprised. In some cases, the supplements I recommend may not make sense. For instance, until Jelly-Kids comes out with a teen and adult formula, I recommend taking two doses of the children's pack, a safe and effective way to get a multivitamin. And, since you need to eat anyway, and it is best to get your vitamins and minerals through food for better absorption, I sometimes suggest grabbing a sport bar and/or beverage in lieu of a meal because it's easy, portable and you get extra vitamin D and minerals. You even get some trace minerals, often more difficult to find in whole foods on a regular basis.

However, in some cases, it's just plain old easier to consume and carry. An updated list of supplements will be available from time-to-time so check _www.thetropicaldiet.com_ website for these updates.

Athlete Supplement Recommendations*

Vitamin or mineral	Product	Dosage**
Multivitamin	_Jelly-Kids_™	1-2 packs daily, morning, and evening
Protein and vitamins & Minerals	PowerBar® ProteinPlus™ sugar free bar EAS™ _AdvantEdge_®	1 bar for snack or 1 beverage per day
Antioxidants	Twinlab _Radical Fighters_	1 pill after workout
B-vitamins	_Twinlab_® _Stress B-Complex Caps_	1 pill in the evening, or 1 before/after drinking alcoholic beverages
Calcium, vitamin D, K	_Viactiv_® Chews	2 chews/day with meals (1 chew in A.M. 1 chew in P.M.)
Electrolytes and Vitamins or low energy moments	_Emer'gen-C_®	1 packet _in heat,_ in water bottle, 1 time/day _as needed_

*Can also be applied to other _L.A.B._ plans.
**These dosages are not suitable for all people at all times. Please check with your physician or registered dietitian (RD) before consuming any supplements.

4. WHAT ABOUT FLUIDS?

Drink, drink, drink.

From the very first chapter of this book I've talked to you about getting enough fluids to drink. Yes, water is essential for health, sport, and life. You need a minimum of four pints of water on The Tropical Diet—about eight cups a day. You will definitely need more fluids if you exercise, sweat, or live in a hot climate since you can lose up to two liters a day in sweat under these conditions. It only takes your body a 1% fluid loss to wreak havoc and feel listless. More than that 1% loss and get ready. You can even pass out!

While water does not give us calories, it helps us to process, digest, and metabolize the food we eat, use, and expend during all our daily activities including sleep.

Getting enough fluids helps us to:

• Transport nutrients in the blood.
• Assist chemical reactions in the body.
• Protect our joints and spinal chord.
• Lubricate the digestive tract.
• Regulate body temperature.

About 60% of your body is water. Even the dry portions like bone, muscle and teeth are 20%, 75%, and 10% water, respectively. Three places in the body where water resides are:

• Inside the cells as intracellular fluid.
• Outside the cells primarily in blood as extracellular fluid.
• Between the cells, called interstitial fluid.

The body manages how much water is in these compartments by maintaining control over the protein, carbohydrates, and fat, as well as the electrolytes, minerals like sodium, chloride and potassium found inside and outside the cells.

Fluid Needs

We need lots of water on a daily basis since we lose a lot through sweating, respiration, and urination. You can actually lose close to 1 to 2 liters per day just in your urine, even more if you drink too much alcohol or caffeinated beverages. If you're an athlete training in the heat, you can easily lose ten times that amount.

The rule of thumb for fluid needs is estimated at 9 to 12 cups per day, however Tropical Dieters get lots of fluid more easily than others since the food choices alone contain 75 to 100% fluid in their natural state. Therefore, the more tropical fruits and vegetables you consume, the more likely you will be able to get away with less actual drinking liquid. Just take a look at the fluid content of tropical foods in Table 4.

But don't throw away the water bottle yet. Fill it up with some bottled water, green, oolong, or black iced tea, Gatorade, Accelerade,100% fruit juice, or any other tasty drink. You can even get away with caffeinated beverages like tea and diet soda just as long as it does not take the place of more nutritious beverages or fluid-rich tropical foods over time.

Table 4
Fluid Content of Tropical Fruits, Vegetables, and Foods*

90% or more fluid

Lemon, cucumber, celery, endive, lettuce, radish, cabbage, spaghetti squash, chayote, soy milk, cauliflower, watermelon, strawberry, tomato, chives, asparagus, tomatillo, eggplant, turnip, red bell pepper, papaya, carambola, spinach, alfalfa sprouts, mushroom, grapefruit, broccoli, melon, okra, bean sprouts, scallions

80-89%

Peach, beet, winter squash, cantaloupe, lemon, onion, passion fruit, lime, tangerine, mandarin orange, carrot, orange, pineapple, apricot, cranberry, brussel sprouts, raspberry, pear, cherry, guava, jicama, blackberries, plum, apple, artichoke, quince, kiwi, leek, lychee, pomegranate, prickly pear, persimmon, shallot, blueberry, avocado, grapes, mango

70-79%

Fresh fig, sapodilla, pear, peas, banana, cherimoya, water chestnut, avocado, sweet potato, jackfruit, yam

60-69%

Beans, lentils, tofu, corn, cassava, malaga, plantain, chickpea

---

Fluid Content of Tropical Fruits, Vegetables, and Foods* (cont'd)

50-59%

Garlic, tempeh

Less than 50%

Nuts, dried fruits, prune, peach, fig, date, raisin

———————

* Water content may vary due to harvest and ripeness of food

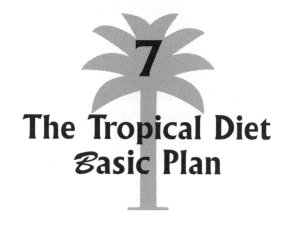

The Tropical Diet
Basic Plan

Picture yourself sitting down to a lean strip steak, drizzled with a vodka-spiked steak sauce, coupled with a side of crisp salad greens dressed with a tangy raspberry vinaigrette, a full-bodied glass of merlot and a rich chocolate spa brownie for dessert. Yes, this can be yours and more on the Tropical Diet Basic program.

Is this your first dietary vacation? Not really sure how to dress or what to do while ashore? Maybe you've been on this trip before, e.g. the lose 10 pounds, gain 20 pounds back plan. Well, climb on board . . . the Basic program may be the plan you've been looking for to get a grasp on a few healthy eating and lifestyle tips that will help you lose some weight and get into shape without losing all the fun in your life. It's also the lover's plan, the romantic side of healthy eating on The Tropical Diet program.

The *Basic* program is a balanced plan of protein, fats, and carbohydrates for dieters who want to maintain a balanced diet or just do best losing weight with 40% carbohydrates/30% protein/ 30% fat, similar to *Zone™-style* eating programs. A balance of carbohydrates, proteins, and fats at every meal may help these dieters manage their appetites, blood sugars, and satiety levels on this style of eating. First-time dieters, those who have been ordered by their doctors to lose a few pounds for health reasons, do well with this program since it has the most fat, flexibility and the most fun out of all three *L.A.B.* programs. You get approximately 30% of total calories in fat, the least amount of carbohydrates with 43 to 45% of total calories, and a handsome balance of meats, chicken, pork, poultry, fish, and eggs as protein sources out of all three plans.

The advantages of a *B*asic eating program are:

- Better maintenance of blood sugar levels than with high-carbohydrate programs.
- A larger portion of protein and fat to help satiate and control hunger levels.
- Easy-to-prepare meals. In fact, you can even order *Zone™-style* meals to go!
- Easy-to-find restaurants which serve a variety of foods that can meet this plan's guidelines.
- Easy-to-cook for others while adhering to this plan since balance of all food groups is allowed.

As with any dietary program, there are always some drawbacks to any specific eating regimen. For this plan, they can include:

- More rigidity than the other *L.A.B.* plans since a stricter adherence to meal calories of less than 500 calories for meals and 100 calories for snacks is advised with a more rigid distribution of calories at each meal into the 40/30/30 carbohydrate, protein, and fat regimen is recommended.
- A need for alcohol discipline and portion control since this is the only plan in which alcohol is included on a regular basis and may contribute to many side effects. Although a direct connection is weak, alcoholic beverages do provide a calorie-dense, nutrient poor energy source which may contribute to obesity.
- Insufficient carbohydrates for athletes who train aerobically (Chapter 6), more than 2 hours each day.
- The difficulty of fat control especially when eating out since fats is included at all mealtimes. However, the program builds in a "fat buffer," to keep dieters within the 30% total fat guideline.

The Basic Phytochemical Boost

The major difference between this *Basic* plan and any other 40/30/30 program is how you will learn to dress up your everyday meals with some of the magical nutrients you may have not even realized existed that you can use to enhance the nutritional value of your meals. These ingredients are called phytochemicals.

Phytochemicals are just what they sound like. Phyto is the Greek word for plants, which describes the nonessential nutrients found within thousands of plant-based foods. These chemical compounds help prevent the formation of cancer-causing compounds called carcinogens, may shrink tumors and may prevent the regrowth of cancerous tumors, and block the enzymes that transform harmless chemicals into carcinogens. Phytochemicals can even act as "antioxidants," like vitamins C, E, and beta-carotene can protect the cells of the body from destructive "free radicals" agents which attack our body's cells and cause us to wrinkle, age, or develop a chronic illness. These chemicals may even help to lower your cholesterol levels and limit your heart disease risk.

Tropical Diet foods, fruits, and vegetables, are loaded with phytochemicals. Foods and herbs with the highest anti-cancer properties include garlic, soybeans, cabbage, ginger, licorice, carrots, celery, cilantro, parsley, and parsnips. Modest levels are found in onions, flax, citrus, turmeric, cruciferous vegetables, tomatoes, and peppers, brown rice, and whole wheat. Other foods with some mild activity are oats, barley, mint, rosemary, thyme, oregano, sage, basil, cucumber, cantaloupe, and berries.

If possible, the key is to add these foods and spices to every meal. Many of the foods and other phytochemical-rich foods are included in almost every Tropical Diet recipe and on all the menus. The following table lists the specific names of the Tropical Diet phyto-rich foods and their health benefits.

Tropical Diet Phyto-Rich Foods
and their Potential Health Benefits

Food/Phytochemical	Health Benefit
Garlic, onions, leeks, chives *allylic sulfides*	may stimulate enzymes which detoxify carcinogens
Hot peppers *capsaicin*	may prevent carcinogens from binding to DNA
Tomatoes (red pigment in other fruits and vegetables) *lycopene*	antioxidant
Tomatoes, strawberries and Pineapple *chlorogenic acid*	may prevent carcinogenic molecules from binding to cells
Berries *ellagic acid*	may neutralize carcinogens
Soy products *flavonoids* *phytosterols* *genistein*	may keep cancer-causing hormones from latching onto a cell receptor site; (prevents tumors from developing and becoming solid; and possibly reduces cholesterol
Green and black tea *polyphenols* *flavonoids*	antioxidant
Avocados and watermelon glutathione	antioxidant
Cruciferous vegetables *indoles* *sulforaphane*	stimulates enzymes that make estrogen less effective, possibly reducing cancer risk; may reduce stomach, colon, and breast cancers by triggering an enzyme to transport carcinogens out of the cell

Food/Phytochemical	Health Benefit
Citrus fruits *limonene*	may shrink tumors and prevent regrowth
Strawberries, pineapple and **bell peppers** *P-couramic acid*	may prevent binding of potentially carcinogenic molecules made during protein digestion
Grains *phenols*	may prevent carcinogens from reacting with target sites
phytates	may deactivate potent hormones that lead to tumor growth
Grapes *resveratrol* *flavonoids* *quercetin*	may inhibit tumor growth; anti-inflammatory anticlotting properties antioxidant
Tea *tannins*	may prevent carcinogens from reacting with target sites
Oranges and eggplant *terpenes*	may produce enzymes that deactivate carcinogens

*B*asic Plan Menus

The *B*asic plan menus differ from the *L*ean and *A*thlete plan menus, because there is a greater emphasis on the even distribution of protein, fat, and carbohydrates at each meal and snack. And while all the *L*ean plan choices work on these menus, the high-carbohydrate *A*thlete plan choices do not. High-glycemic index (page 100) carbohydrates are not recommended. Many of the starch-based entrees from the *A*thlete plan are not suitable for this program. Think of your plate divided into three portions with a greater emphasis on the protein, a thumbnail or two of oil or fat, a healthy portion of colorful vegetables, and a small helping of sliced tropical fruits.

Calories	1200	1500	1800	2000
Food Groups:				
Milk	2 cup	2 cups	2 cups	3 cups
Fruit	4 fruits	5 fruits	6 fruits	6 fruits
Vegetables	2 cups	2 cups	2 cups	3 cups
Grains	2	3	4	4
Protein	8 oz.	10 oz.	12 oz.	14 oz.
Fat	5 tsp.	6 tsp.	8 tsp.	8 tsp.

The Basic Guide to Meals

Here is your guide to meal planning. The key to eating the Basic-style diet is to emphasize a balance of carbohydrate, protein, and fats at all meals and snacks. Additional Basic menu choices can be found in Chapter 8.

Meals	Food Servings	Examples
Breakfast	2 protein servings or 1 dairy	egg white omelette or fat free yogurt
	1 fruit	½ c. mixed berries with
	1 fat	sunflower seeds
Snack	1 protein or 1 fat	1 low fat string cheese
		1 oz. soy nuts
Lunch	3 to 4 protein	4 oz. chicken sub
	1 to 2 cups vegetables	with lettuce/tomato
	1 fat	1 tbsp. mayonnaise
		on whole grain bread

Meals	Food Servings	Examples
Snack	2 fruits 1 protein	berry smoothie with protein powder supplement scoop or trail mix
Dinner	1 cup vegetables 3 to 4 protein 2 starch 1 fat	1 cup minestrone soup 3 to 4 oz. grilled salmon ½ c. yellow rice 1 tsp. oil for tossed salad dressing or for alcoholic beverage

The best way to add a tropical twist is to garnish the dishes with tropical fruits, fresh steamed vegetables, or to season your dish with a dab of Tabasco sauce, hot sauce, ginger, curry, or fresh herbs like mint, parsley, basil, or cilantro.

A Day in the Life of the *Basic Plan Dieter*

On this plan, you will get to eat more meat including exotic meat like game, fatty fish such as salmon and mackerel, dressing on your salads, cheese on your lunch wrap, and dessert. Trail mix, guacamole with baked chips, and cheese with apple slices for a snack are just some of the typical snacks you will have to choose from.

Here is a typical day in the life of the *Basic* eater:

Breakfast:
1 grapefruit half, seasoned with fresh mint
Egg white omelette with low-fat cheese and green veggies, onion, and yellow pepper
½ cup of Tropicana® Lite orange juice
1 cup of java with lite cream

Snack
Apple with 1 oz. low-fat cheese "sauce" melted for dipping

Lunch
6-inch whole-wheat sub sandwich with turkey, lite mayo, lettuce, tomato, pepper and onions

Snack
Guacamole dip with raw veggies such as carrots, celery, and jicama

Dinner
1 glass merlot wine
Green salad, cherry tomatoes, and raspberry vinaigrette
Pan-fried strip steak drizzled with *Imperia* vodka sauce, served with sautéed broccoli and corn
Baked quince spiced with island cinnamon

End-of-the-Chapter Questions

1. WHAT COMPONENTS ARE CRITICAL TO AFFECTING THE WAY MY BODY USES CALORIES?

Three major factors contribute to your calorie needs and ultimately the success of your weight loss and weight maintenance program. They are food choices—the type, amount, and preparation methods, your daily fitness routine—how much, what, and when you exercise, and your mind *metabolism*—how you believe and perceive your body is using calories and the way you visualize your program at work.

Specific foods can impact this weight loss trilogy more than any other factor.

And while all your favorite food choices can fit into your *L.A.B.* plan, there are better food choices you can make at specific times of the day which will improve your caloric efficiency and enhance the quality of your diet. Tropically delicious, high-fiber, vitamin, and mineral-rich foods, hot and spicy foods, and caffeinated products have all been shown to influence the rate your body uses calories, in other words, your metabolism. The impact on your metabolism can be as little as 100 calories or as much as 500 calories each day. You see, not all foods are created equal.

The process of digestion, absorption, and assimilation after eating also requires energy. Five to 30% of the calories you eat will be used for these processes. Collectively, these are known as the SDA, the specific dynamic action of food. You learned how to add or subtract this 10% of total calories in the last chapter.

The nutritional composition of your diet can also influence the calorie-burning capacity during and up to 1 hour after meals. Research has shown that protein can increase your metabolism by 20 to 30% and this can last up to 3 to 5 hours.

High-fat diets of 59% total calories or more have been associated with reduced energy expenditure. That means for the same amount of calories, fattier foods cause more stored body fat than carbohydrate-rich or protein-rich foods. Since fat is not typically used as your primary energy source, excessive amounts will cause an accumulation of excess body fat.

Quantity and dietary composition may also influence how many calories you burn each day. To burn more calories, it is better to eat more meals and snacks each day than one huge meal, even if the total calories are the same. So grazing style turns out to be a better calorie burner. However it is not practical for everyone, so my advice is to include as many nibbles as you can throughout the day without going overboard. If in doubt, follow your menu plan.

Now if you're worried about the weekend, holiday, or birthday binges, relax. Contrary to popular belief, the truth is that a once-in-a-while overeating episode will also increase your calorie burn significantly. So don't throw in the towel if you mess up your plan for a day. And while I am not giving you permission to overeat, don't panic or perceive yourself as a failure. It's normal to want to rebel and break the diet once in a while. Just forgive yourself, detox for a day or two, and start your plan all over again.

Undereating, on the other hand will definitely depress your body's calorie-burning capacity. Research has shown that those who fast or self-impose a starvation, such as in anorexia nervosa, can cause a sluggish metabolism. This is a built-in mechanism from the *Mighty One* to protect us from breaking down during fasting periods, starvation, or while adhering to low-calorie diets.

This automatic "gear" actually dates back to the beginning of time when cave people would have a lot of food and then go for periods without food. This adaptive mechanism has been described in other programs. This metabolic "pacer" can also be seen in endurance athletes like marathon runners and Ironman triathletes. It is designed to preserve calories for intense exercise sessions and/or recovery periods.

One last note on the eating to burn topic.

If binging or undereating or any unusual dieting or eating behaviors become a familiar pattern, then you may need to seek extra help from your Tropical Diet nutritionist, or a psychotherapist to look at other issues that may be affecting your success in food, fitness, and in life.

2. SO WHAT ABOUT ALCOHOL? SHOULD I OR SHOULDN'T I HAVE A DAILY BREW, GLASS OF WINE OR HARD ALCOHOLIC BEVERAGE?

Research suggests a moderate daily alcohol intake may actually have a beneficial effect on health. How much is moderate? A moderate intake of alcohol in my opinion is all relative although some experts have agreed on a specific amount. In my opinion, a moderate amount is one drink, equal to a 12 oz. beer, 4 oz. of wine, or 1.5 oz. 80 proof liquor.

However, this is where I draw the line and ask, what is moderate for you? Can you handle a drink on a daily basis or if you have a drink one day, do you need more the next day and even more alcohol over time. You know if you're the type of individual who has an alcohol problem if you can't control your moods, behaviors, or emotions after a drink or two. However, it's ultimately up to you, your family, and physician to determine if drinking alcohol is right for you or not.

Case in point. I love alcohol.

To me alcoholic beverages are tasty, creative, fun, social to drink, enjoy and consume and downright delicious when added to sauces, stir-fries, and desserts. I have been enjoying alcoholic beverages almost my entire adult life with the exception of 6 years while I was competing professionally in triathlon, wanting nothing to interfere with my potential to be my personal best.

Fast forward to 40.

When I turned 40, alcohol turned sour on me. For some reason, and I'm not sure whether it's medical, emotional, or physical, alcohol is not making me feel happy and giddy anymore. Maybe it's a period, maybe its pre-pre-pre-pre menopause, although I have had no tests to show that I am close to that stage in life outside my age (and I do the girl thing like clockwork.) I just can't figure it out, but alcohol, whether it is a glass of wine or champagne with dinner, a cold brew by the pool during the hot Miami summer, or a liqueur to satisfy my sweet craving after dinner, does not work for me right now.

It makes me tired, depressed, and downright unsocial. I decided on my 40th New Years Eve to give up alcohol. Ouch!

Despite not being a heavy drinker, I had to detox from the habit of going for a drink with company, at sporting events or on vacation. It was tough at times, but now I am really glad I made the choice because I feel great and am back to competing again at the national level.

If you do choose to drink alcohol, I feel obliged to offer you the following information, particularly if you choose to participate in sports.

Point #1. Muscles cannot use alcohol as an energy source, and is eventually stored as fat. *So if you drink too much, even as you watch your calorie intake, you can become fat.*

Point #2. While the body is processing alcohol, it limits the amount of sugar it releases to the bloodstream. This causes hypoglycemia (low blood sugar) and fatigue. *This means when you drink alcohol, it will limit your ability to feel energized and may even increase your appetite.*

Point #3. Drinking alcohol may also contribute to hypothermia during cold weather. *If you live in a cold climate, a nice warm cider by the fireplace can actually make you colder in the long run.*

Point #4. Consuming alcohol can also lead to indigestion, nausea and vomiting, muscle, heart, brain, and esophagus abnormalities and liver damage. *Need I say more? Watch the quantities you consume.*

Point #5 Alcohol, like caffeine acts as a diuretic causing increased urination and water loss. To metabolize 1 ounce of alcohol the body requires 8 ounces water. *That means you need to drink a minimum of 1 glass of water with every alcoholic drink you consume or, drink a mixed drink like vodka and orange juice. You'll even get an antioxidant boost with each drink (See* *Nutrition Bite on The Imperia Vodka story.)*

Point #6. B-vitamins are required to process alcohol therefore limiting their use for carbohydrate, protein, and fat metabolism. *If you choose to drink, take an extra B-vitamin before your late night out so you buffer the system with extra Bs to handle the alcoholic load.*

Point #7. If you have a family history of alcoholism, substance abuse, or domestic violence, alcohol may not be for you. *There are plenty of alcohol-free beers, wines, and beverages for those who choose not to drink or cannot handle alcohol.*

If you do choose to indulge in drinking, here are some additional tips.

- Drink one-cup fortified water like Propel® for every alcoholic drink consumed to prevent the effects of dehydration and B-vitamin depletion.
- Get extra B-vitamins in your diet either with a pre-drinking supplement or by consuming the *brown* diet, e.g., lean meat, pork, chicken, turkey, pretzels, bean dip, or fortified bars or beverages.
- Beer and wine also gives you additional carbs. When you drink beer, subtract 2 servings of starch or bread from your daily diet. If you have a 4 oz. glass of wine, subtract 2 fruit servings.
- Don't skip healthy meals to consume booze. Eat fresh fruits, salads, lean meats, and lowfat dairy during the day, so if the booze causes a missed evening meal, at least you got your nutrients for the day. Also fortify your diet with a multivitamin. I like Jelly-Kids™, new on the market, easy to consume and stick in your pocket since it's individually packaged. It's really a kid's multivitamin, so you can even have two packages and it'll be safe to consume.
- Finally, don't drink the night before a road or airplane trip, competition or turning-point professional job interview, meeting, or presentation. Drinking alcohol tends to mess up your good intentions the next day. Think about it. You normally need more fluids, decent meals, and lots of rest the day after a drinking event. Drink only when you have the time to recover properly the night after.

3. I'VE HEARD THE SAME ABOUT CAFFEINE. IS IT OKAY FOR ME TO HAVE A MORNING AFTERNOON, OR EVEN AN EVENING EXPRESSO? I'VE BEEN DRINKING COFFEE SINCE I'VE BEEN IN MY TEENS WITHOUT ANY PROBLEMS.

The risks and benefits of caffeine are a curse and blessing all in one cup.

There is no doubt we get going after our morning brew, both psychologically and physiologically. If it weren't for a hit of iced tea, dict soda, or a sugar-free energy drink first thing in the morning, it would have been nearly impossible for me to train hard 4 to 7 mornings a week for the past 20 years when I need to start my exercise before 5 A.M. to beat the tropical morning heat. Caffeine lifts your spirit in the morning, afternoon, or evening. It keeps us going to tend to work, school, and family responsibilities. It is a tradition to stop for a morning café con leche or *Café Cubaño*, the Latin version of brew in the tropics.

Caffeine works by dilating our blood vessels, and by bringing more oxygen to muscles. It actually helps speed up your metabolism by encouraging sugars and fats in your blood to get used for energy. It also helps to rev up our adrenaline engines, our competitive response hormone, which prepares us for competition and for life's work.

There are long-term health benefits too.

Research has shown that caffeine can:
• Stimulate our metabolism and help us burn more calories during the day.
• Help us burn more fat calories.
• Decrease body fat.
• Lower low-density lipoproteins (LDL), the bad cholesterol in hypercholesterolemic adults.
• Lower risk for late onset diabetes.
• Possibly help prevent symptomatic gallstone disease.

As with anything else that makes you feel good, there are drawbacks to consuming too much caffeine. Some of the side effects include heart palpitations, nervousness, poor sleep, and diarrhea, but these can vary from person to person. Chronic caffeine consumption can cause painful, lumpy breasts called fibrocystic breast disease and has been linked to elevated blood cholesterol and premenstrual syndrome (PMS).

So what is my best advice to you?

• If you have any of the negative symptoms associated with caffeine consumption, limit your intake to 1 cup in the morning or the minimal amount necessary just to get your day started.
• Don't drink it in the evenings if you find you are not sleeping soundly.
• Drink oolong or green tea for additional phytochemical benefits.
• Find out which of your beverages and foods have caffeine and

limit yourself to one serving a day. Foods and beverages which include caffeine are tea, and chocolate foods like candy, sport bars, pops and cocoa, as well as decongestants also typically contain caffeine.

TROPICAL
FOOD SCIENCE

Part III

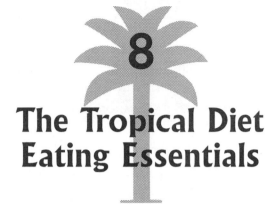

The Tropical Diet
Eating Essentials

This is the fun part of the book, especially for those of you who like to get practical food tips. Now is the time you get to shop—stock up on the foods you will need for your Tropical Diet eating plan.

This chapter simulates the Caribbean cruise experience. In this case, you get to visit your Tropical Diet ports-of-call—your food and ingredient needs over the next few weeks. Your itinerary is your kitchen, local grocery store, health food store, ethnic or gourmet grocery store, and local restaurants. Practical food tips, shopping lists, your Tropical Diet Kitchen staple list, menus, and eating-out guide can all be found on the pages to follow.

Before you head out on your chapter's adventure, ignite an exciting food experience as you establish your Tropical Diet kitchen.

Celebrate your new dietary journey with a new eating ambiance. Go ahead and treat yourself to a few new household goods to set the tropical mood of your dining area. Purchase a few colorful, fresh or faux flower arrangements. Pick up some brightly colored placemats to brighten up your meals. Add a freshly ground pepper and salt mill to the table. And for a real island setting, get yourself a bottle of a Caribbean spice that's never missing from the table—a bottle of hot sauce to rev up your mood, metabolism, and dieting spirit!

And for a romantic touch, dress up your table with some candlestick holders. There's nothing more romantic than eating by candlelight to soft music regardless of what's on the menu— whether you're eating fast food or gourmet cuisine.
Celebrate the moment. Your time has arrived.

Tropical Diet Kitchen Foundation Food List Pantry Staples

This is a list of all the necessary ingredients you should try to have on hand in one way, shape or another to be prepared to cook a gourmet meal or whip out a dish at the drop of a hat. While fresh is always best, do not feel pressured to buy fresh only. If you walk into my home, you will find a balance of fresh with canned and frozen. In fact, research has shown that in some cases canned and frozen can be just as nutritious as fresh. And as we all know, frozen and canned foods have a better shelf life and are much more economical.

Vegetables
Deep green leafy vegetables, canned also
    acceptable
Broccoli
Red, yellow, and green peppers
Tomato and tomato products
Chayote
Beets, fresh or canned salt free

Also acceptable:
Frozen, unsalted vegetables—single or mixed
    selections—store brand acceptable
Canned, organic, and/or salt free

Fruits
Oranges
Pink grapefruit
Kiwi
Blueberries
Strawberries

Mango
Pineapple
Watermelon
Pear
Apple

Also acceptable
Frozen unsweetened blueberries, strawberries,
    and mixed fruit
Canned fruits in their own juice
100% fruit juice

Grains/starchy vegetables
Sweet potato
Middle Eastern couscous
Papadini lentil pasta
Pastato Fortified Pasta
Barbara's Mashed potatoes
Frozen and/or fresh peas and corn

Grains/starchy vegetables (cont'd)
Fresh, Canned, or frozen beans, lentils
Glenny's® or GeniSoy® Soy Crisps
Goldmine Mungbean Chips
Pupadoms Crackers
Elephant spring roll wrappers

Protein
Fresh eggs
Eggology egg whites
Boneless chicken breasts
Gimme Lean protein Substitute
Caribbean Tofu
Pink salmon
Lean pork
PowerBar ProteinPlus sugar-free apple
    caramel bar
Primal Spirit® Foods Primal Soy Strips
EAS AdvantEdge Carb Control Shake-1.5
    protein servings

Dairy
Dannon Light n' Fit Smoothie in tropical,
    peach passion or mixed berries
Land O Lakes fat free half & half
Sargento Fat Free Cheddar and Mozzarella
    Cheese
Lactaid fat-free milk

Fats
Fresh avocado
Whole unsalted almonds
Whole unsalted walnuts
Roasted soy nuts
Sunflower seeds
Barlean's Forti Flax Ground flaxseed
Soy Wonder® nut butter
Smuckers® Baking Healthy™ oil and
    shortening replacement*

Land O Lakes Fat Free half and half
I Can't Believe It's Not Butter Spray*

Beverages
Propel flavored waters
Arizona infused waters
Syfo sugar-free fruit flavored seltzers
Tropicana Essentials Light and Healthy
    orange juice
FUZE™ Tropical Punch Slenderize
Rocamojo™ Blend Coffee+
Myoplex Carb Sense French Vanilla Drink
EAS-AdvantEdge low-carb drink—vanilla,
    chocolate or strawberry
Gatorade Tropical Flavor Sports Drink—
    A plan
Accelerade Sports and Recovery drink—
    A plan
H_2 COCO® 100% coconut water
Boost® Breeze™ Tropical Fruit flavored drink

Sport Bars/Products
Meyers Squib
PowerBar
Luna® Tropical Crisp Bar
Tropical Fruit flavored Power gel

Seasoning/spice
Fresh is best when possible
Basil
Cilantro/culantro
Ginger
Parsley
Kosher Salt
Black pepper
Seitenbacher® instant all-natural, gluten-free
    vegetable broth mix

Sweets

Fruitfull® lowfat frozen fruit pops

Heavenly Desserts™ Sugar Free, Fat Free
Meringue

Fat Free, sugar free hot chocolate

No Pudge® fat-free fudge brownie mix

Aunt Gussie's Fat free sugar free Orange
Biscottini

Sharkies® Organic Energy Fruit Chews—
A plan

Miss Meringue classic Meringue cookies—
FREE

10 CarboLITE gummy bears—1 fruit serving,
0 net carbs

Haagen Daz® Mango Sorbet

---

*Fat-free substitute

+Has 7 grams protein and half the caffeine of regular coffee. Also available in decaf.

The Tropical Diet Food List

This list is your *tropical food bible*, your guide to finding out where your favorite foods fit, how much you can eat, and what tropical nutrients they contain based on the food's content.

As you can imagine, there are hundreds of foods and combinations of foods you can eat on a daily basis. That's why I have provided a restaurant-type menu for your four weeks of dieting since your personal eating habits, lifestyle, and schedule will dictate how you consume your daily *L.A.B.* plan.

Please understand that while most of the foods can be found at any national or local large grocery chain, many foods may look strange to you if you've never walked into a health food store, natural market, ethnic, or gourmet grocery or even online at Melissa's, Frieda's, or Robert is Here websites. Don't let that deter you. Let it encourage you to fantasize about all the menu possibilities available to you.

The foods are listed according to specific portion sizes based on their food category and dietary composition. For instance, in the milk/dairy equivalent food group, drinking 1 cup of skim milk would be the same as consuming 6-oz. of low-fat yogurt. In the meat and protein food group, a 3-oz. hamburger would be the same as selecting a 6-oz. can of tuna. Of course, there are vitamin and mineral differences between foods. Fiber and phytochemical content also vary between food choices. However, when it comes down to the caloric value of each food—the protein, carbohydrate, and fat content of every choice in the group—they are closely related.

These lists standardize the amounts of calories, carbohydrates, proteins, and fats of the six major food groups: milk, protein, vegetables, grains, fruits, and fats. The Tropical Diet version of these food lists highlight the most nutritious Tropical Diet food choices for each food group and emphasize the products made with tropical ingredients. Over 100 foods are represented on the lists. Updates to the list can be found at the website *www.thetropicaldiet.com.*

The Tropical Diet Food Groups can be compared to other food exchange—type programs like the Weight Watchers food lists and the American Diabetes, and Dietetic Association's Food Lists for Meal Planning designed for individuals with diabetes, hypoglycemia, weight, and other medically related challenges. Therefore, if there are other non-tropically-related frozen, fast, or convenient foods you desire, they can be easily worked into the program. On The Tropical Diet, your choices are unlimited and universal.

The food groups listed are: proteins and meat alternatives, dairy and its substitutes, vegetables, fruits, fats, and grains/starches. The calorie, carbohydrate, protein, and fat content from each group can be found in the charts on page 266–269.

The lists of foods also include The Tropical Diet recipes in the book and their food group nutritional breakdowns.

How to use these lists:

1. Take the Tropical Diet Taste Test to find out your best Tropical Diet *L.A.B.* Plan.
2. Find your personal plan in Chapters 5 through 7. Your program's chapter will show you the number of portions you can eat from each food group on a daily basis.
3. Build your pantry with my Tropical Diet food choices listed in the food foundation list in Chapter 8.
4. Follow your food program as closely as the book suggests for nutritional adequacy and dietary success.
5. Keep track of your dietary success with The Tropical Diet Pocket Coach©.
6. Make a variety of selections each day in order to achieve your optimal nutritional intake.

7. Use the menus to help you to stick to your plan when you are unsure about the foods you need to eat, how to prepare them, and how often to eat them.

You can also eat your personal favorite foods on the program after two weeks of successful Tropical Diet eating. Check the nutritional analysis of the food on the label or send the recipe to the *www.thetropicaldiet.com* website for an free nutritional analysis.

You can also take a shot at analyzing your recipe yourself. Just take a look at the food label for the food you want to eat, fit it into the appropriate food category, check the serving size, fit the best portion size of your food into the guidelines of the food group and voila . . . you've performed your own analysis.

For instance, if your food is a frozen fruit pop, with 100 calories per pop it is a fruit-type food that exceeds the fruit portion size by 40 calories. That means when you eat one of these fruit pops, you've had close to two servings of fruits from your fruit allotment for the day. Let's say you have 4 fruit servings to "spend" each day, you have used half of your fruit servings. That's okay. The food fits on your daily program. However, choosing a frozen fruit pop on a regular basis will give you more sugar and less fiber, phytochemicals, vitamins and minerals than a piece of fresh fruit so it's best not to use all your fruit servings for a pop. However, if you do, it's not the end of the world. It works.

Let's take another example. You've created a delicious tropical chicken salad with a fruit variation. You want to know the analysis so you log onto *www.thetropicaldiet.com* website and find out one portion has 3 oz. protein, 1 cup of vegetables, and 3 servings of fruit. What you then do is subtract the amount of food serving from each of your daily totals to account for the amount you have consumed at your meal or snack. And while you may have lots of room for your specialty chicken salad on your personal program, as with all successful dieting, planning is key. Preparing for your 3 protein, 3 fruit dish will help you balance the rest of the day with foods from other groups. This is how you lose weight now and keep it off for the long run.

TROPICAL DIET PROTEIN SERVINGS

Analysis per serving:
80 calories, 7-10 grams protein, and variable fat

1 oz. chicken, turkey, lean beef, ham, or pork

1 egg (add one fat serving)

5 egg whites

2 oz. shellfish

2 oz. fish (see recommended list)

2 oz. water-packed tuna

2 oz. Lifeline® Jalapeno Jack, Swiss or other flavored fat-free cheeses

1 oz. low-fat cheese

¼ cup Light 'n Lively® or Breakstone® fat-free cottage cheese (snack size)

¾ cup egg whites

Tropical Fish

Mahi Mahi

Swordfish

Grouper

Tuna

Red snapper

Sushi*

Maki (1 slice = approx. ½ starch, ½ protein)

1 cone sushi†(1 starch, 1 protein)

Protein alternatives

1 low fat veggie burger

4 oz. seitan

2 oz. Soy Boy® Caribean tofu (1 fat*)

6 oz. lite tofu

2 oz. fat-free Soya Kaas® cheese

2 oz. Gimme Lean® Meatless ground meat

¼ cup TVP

1 Primal Strip® "jerky" (1½ protein, ½ fat)**

1 cup Rocamojo™ Coffee (1 protein)

---

*deduct this (serving) from the other food category listed

**available from:

Northern Soy, Inc.

545 West Ave, Westchester, New York, 14611-2497

†Sushi source-Ann Litt, RD, author of *The College Student's Guide to Eating Well on Campus*

◉▮ Nutrition Nugget

To Eat Fish or Not, That is the Question
Farmed or Wild Fish . . . Which one is healthier?

Nutritionally speaking, farmed and wild fish are similar in protein, vitamins and minerals. Farmed fish tends to be higher in total fat since they don't get much swimming exercise! The omega-3 content in both types of fish are similar.

Fatty fish like salmon will also accumulate more toxins like PCBs and mercury even if they are farmed. Antibiotics and other drugs can leave a residue in the fish.

Best Choices?
• Alaskan salmon and halibut, mahi mahi, bluefish, and fluke. Almost all canned salmon is Alaskan.
• Farmed shellfish like oysters, scallops, and clams.
• Catfish, trout, and tilapia raised onshore are less harmful to the environment.
• Wild Alaskan salmon is preferred over domestic or imported but is very expensive.
• Ecofish, ecologically safe seafood sold at Wild Oats and other markets.

Unhealthy choices?
• Farm-raised shrimp and salmon.
• King mackerel is a larger predatory fish that has more risk of mercury contamination.

Additional information and a "tuna calculator," a tool to help you to calculate your recommended tuna intake can be found at the website *www.ewg.org/issues/mercury/20031209/calculator.php*

TROPICAL DIET DAIRY AND SUBSTITUTES SERVINGS

Analysis per serving:
100 calories, 8 grams protein, 12 grams carbohydrates, variable fat

1 cup Lactaid® nonfat milk
1 cup Lactaid® 1% fat milk (½ fat)

1 Haagen Daz® Frozen Yogurt Bar
covered with Raspberry Sorbet
1 Bottle Dannon® Tropical Fruit Fusion
Smoothie—(1 dairy, 2½ fruits ½ fat)
4 oz. Light 'n Lively® or Breakstone®
snack pack non-fat cottage cheese
1 Yoplait Whips™ Key Lime Pie lowfat
yogurt (½ fruit, ½ fat)
1 Yonique® Guava lowfat yogurt (½
fruit)
1 Yonique® Pina Colada lowfat yogurt
(1 fruit)
1 La Yogurt® Sabor Latino Guava or
Mango (1 fruit)
1 Dan Active™ Drink
1 Yoplait® Nouriche Tropical nonfat
yogurt (1 additional milk, 1.5 fruit
servings)

Substitutes
1 cup soy drink, Fat Free Pacific®
Vanilla*
1 cup Nutrisoy® vanilla low fat soy
milk (½ fat) **
6 oz. soy yogurt
8 oz. small container Stonyfield
Farms™ fat-free yogurt (1.5 milk)
1 cup non-fat Kefir
1 cup White Wave™ chocolate soy
beverage****
1 frozen Tofutti™ treat
1 cup Pacific® rice non-fat cocoa
drink***

---

*deduct this (serving) from other food category
*Pacific Vanilla soy drink is fortified w/ Vitamins A, D and calcium
**Nutrisoy is fortified w/vitamins A, D, B_2, and calcium
***Pacific rice drink is fortified w/ A, D and calcium
****White Wave Silk chocolate soy beverage is fortified with vitamins A, D, B_2, B_{12}, and calcium

TROPICAL DIET FAT SERVINGS
Per serving: approximately 45 calories, 5 grams fat

⅛ medium avocado

1 tbsp. sunflower seeds

2 tbsp. coconut

20 small peanuts

1 tbsp. soy nut butter (2 fat servings)

2 tsp. peanut butter (1.5 fat servings)

1 tsp. margarine or butter

1 tsp. olive, walnut, almond, hazelnut, sunflower, soybean and canola vegetable oil

2 tsp. Pataks curry paste

1.5 tbsp. "Iri Goma" roasted sesame seeds

2 tbsp. IKARI non-oil sesame dressing (*¼ protein)

4 tbsp. Land O Lakes Fat free half & half (½ starch, no fat)

Salad Dressings

1 oz. (2 tbsp.) Miko Key Lime Ginger Dressing and Marinade

Nonfat Dressing

1 oz. (2 tbsp.) Consorzio® Raspberry & Balsamic dressing (1 fruit)

1 oz. Wishbone® Fat Free Ranch Dressing (½ starch)

1 oz. Wishbone® Italian Dressing (⅓ fruit)

◉ Nutrition Nugget

A note about soy nut butter:

Soy nut butter has more protein, 8 grams per serving, and 1.5 grams saturated fat when compared with peanut butter per serving

TROPICAL DIET FRUITS & FRUIT PRODUCTS

Analysis per serving:
60 calories, 15 grams carbohydrates

1 apple, orange, pear, peach, kiwi,
½ banana, mango
1¼ cups strawberries, watermelon
¾ cup pineapple, blueberries
15 grapes
1 cup papaya, raspberries,
½ cup cranberries or rhubarb
1 cup cantaloupe (1/3 melon)
2 plums
¾ cup mandarin oranges

Drinks/juices

1 cup Gatorade®
1 container Vruit Tropical Blend 100%
    Juice (2 fruits)
½ cup orange, apple, grapefruit, or
    pineapple juice
⅓ cup cranberry, prune, or grape juice
4 oz. wine (2 fruits)

Dried Fruits:

4 apple rings
7 apricot halves
2 pieces "Ego" dried guava
2 tbsp. dried cranberries (1½ fruits)
3 pieces Woodstock Farms® ginger
    slices
1 oz. La Vigne® Star Fuyu persimmons
2 figs
1 oz. raisins
1 "Go Banana" or similar dried banana
¼ cup strawberries*
¼ cup blueberries*
3 prunes

Fruit related or other sweet foods

1 Orgran® Banana fruit bar
6 fruit splashed Sharkies® (½ bag—
    1¼ fruits)
1 Dole® reduced sugar Pears in Kiwi-
    berry gel or Papaya in peach gel
1 Stretch Island™ Truly Tropical Fruit
    Leather—1 fruit
1 oz. freeze-dried "Just Fruit
    Munchies" (2 fruits)
1 tbsp. molasses or brown rice syrup
1 tbsp. jam or jelly
3 tbsp. Robert is Here*, all fruit
    Passion Fruit sugar free jam—½ fruit
1 tbsp. Etti banana paste
1 bag Let's Do Organic® Super Sour
    Gummi Bears

---

* ordering information in appendix

TROPICAL DIET VEGETABLES

Analysis *per cup*:
50 calories, 10 grams carbohydrates, 4 grams protein

Eggplant
Broccoli
Kale
Cauliflower
Carrots
Cabbage
Brussel sprouts
Mushrooms
Peppers, red, yellow, orange, green
Okra
Tomatoes
Asparagus
Artichoke
Onions
Squash-zucchini
Radishes
Celery
Mung bean sprouts
Snow peas
Tomato sauce-fat free
Bok choy

Spinach
Collard greens

Other:
Hot "Just Veggies" (½ cup)
1 cup vegetable juice

Sushi*
1 slice vegetable maki (1 slice =
    1½" long = 1 starch)
1 cone vegetable sushi (2 starch)

—————————

* source-Ann Litt, RD, author of *The College Student's Guide To Eating Well on Campus*

TROPICAL DIET GRAINS/STARCHES

Analysis per serving:
80 calories, 15 grams carbohydrates, 2 grams protein, variable fat

Cereals/Grains/pasta

¼ cup Arrowhead Mills™ 4 grain plus Flax Cereal (2 grain servings)

½ cup couscous

3 tbsp. wheat germ

⅓ cup rice

½ cup pasta**

3 tbsp. Grapenuts®

½ cup cooked cereals

½ cup shredded wheat

⅓ cup Lifestream® Smart Bran

½ cup Lifestream® Flax Plus

1 Barbara's Toaster Pastry, like Pop Tart (2 servings grain and ½ fruit)

1 Flax Plus Waffle (1 serving plus ½ protein)

⅔ cup Atkins® Blueberry Bounty cereal with almonds (½ protein)

Bread/Crackers

1 small bag (1.3 oz.) Glenny's® Soy Crisps (2 grain servings)

½ bag Glenny's® apple cinnamon soy crisps

25 GeniSoy® Crisps (1¼ grains)

1 Alvarado Street® sprouted wheat tortilla—(plus ½ protein serving)

1 fat-free flour tortilla (1.5 grain servings)

1 corn tortilla

½ bagel

1 Cracker Flax, apple raisin "crackers" (1.5 grain, 1 fat serving)

7 Japanese "Umenokamaki" Rice Crackers

25 Eden® sea vegetable or wasabi crackers

1 piece JJ Flats™ (1.5 servings)

1 whole wheat pita, small

½ whole wheat pita, large

** Try a variety of pastas including whole wheat spirals, Vita Spelt, Ancient Harvest Quinoa, Sobaya organic wheat and brown rice "soba" pasta, and buckwheat "soba" pasta. Quinoa pasta is rich in B_1, B_2, soba in iron, whole wheat in B_1, B_3

🍽 *Nutrition Nugget*

Glenny's® Soy Crisps

A great healthy snack, one small bag of cheddar cheese snack provides 9 grams of protein, iron, calcium, vitamin D, and K, and folic acid.

TROPICAL DIET GRAINS/STARCHES (cont'd)

Analysis per serving:
80 calories, 15 grams carbohydrates, 2 grams protein, variable fat

Starchy Vegetables
1 baked potato
½ cup mashed potato (Barbara's is organic)
½ cup corn
½ cup peas
⅓ cup yams
¾ cup winter squash (spaghetti, acorn, butternut)

Beans and Bean Products
½ cup Eden's garbanzo beans
½ cup fava or lima beans
⅓ cup pinto beans
1 oz. (2 tbsp.) Fantastic Foods instant hummus (no oil)
¼ cup Fantastic Foods Instant Refried Beans
Shari's refried beans (½ protein)

Chips/snack foods/rice cakes
7 Gold Mine™ Mung Bean and Soybean chips
1 oz. Soken Seaweed crunch crackers (about ½ bag 1½ starch)
8 Baked Lays™
1.5 large rice cakes
8 mini Quaker™ rice cakes
5 Hain™ Mini Rice Cakes
1 large hard Snyder's pretzel (1¼ grains)
7 Shiloh Farms Oat Bran Pretzels
20-23 Cinnamon or plain *Coronilla* Qrunchies, with Quinoa, gluten-free

Other:
3 tsp. arrowroot—½ grain serving
2 tbsp. fat-free ½ and ¼ to ½ starch

Combination Foods
Amy's® black beans, vegetables enchilada 1 package (2 starches, 1 protein)
Amy's® Organic Beans and Rice Burrito (2 grains, ½ protein, 1 fat)
1 slice vegetable maki, 1-1½" slice (1 starch)
1 cone vegetable sushi† (2 starch)

Beverages
1 envelope-sugar free Swiss Miss® Hot Chocolate (1 starch)
1 beer—2 starches
1 lite beer—1½ starches

Sweets
4 Tropical Source® Mango papaya hard candies (1 fruit)
½ Tropical Source® Sundried Jungle banana chocolate bar (1 starch, 1 fruit, 2 fat)
1 bag "Let's Do It . . . Organic" Gummi Bears or Black Licorice Bears (1 starch)
4 pieces Soken Natural Seaweed Candy (1 starch-no simple sugars)
1 Stretch Island Truly Tropical Fruit Leather (1 fruit)
1⅓ tbsp. dark chocolate baking chips, Tropical Source (1 fruit, ½ fat)
3 Kasugai Litchi hard candies (1 fruit)
3 Kasugai Litchi gummy candies (1 fruit)
6 Aunt Gussies Fat Free Sugar Free Orange Biscottini

Sport Bars/Foods and Beverages

1 *Kashi®* Go Lean Sublime Lemon
   Lime Protein and Fiber Bar
   (1 starch, ½ protein, 1 fat)
1 *GeniSoy®* Island Blast Extreme
   Crunch Bar (1 starch, 1 fruit, ½ fat)
1 Luna® Bar Tropical Crisp
   (1 protein, 1 grain, ½ fat)

1 Power Bar® banana (1 starch,
   1 protein, 1 fruit, ½ fat)
1 Sugar-Free PowerBar® Protein Plus™
   caramel apple (1 protein, 1 starch)
1 Clif Bar™—2 starch, 1 fruit, ½ fat
1½ *Sugar Free* Bristol-Meyers Squibb
   Choice, Berry Almond Crispy Bar
1 GU Banana Blitz Energy Gel
   (1¼ starch)

TROPICAL DIET® FREE FOODS

To complement your vegetarian meals, these foods have negligible calories.

Green tea
Lettuce
Garlic
Watercress
Onions
Lemons and limes
Jalapeno
Soy sauce
Mustard
Chili sauce
Salsa
Coffee, tea, or sparkling unsweetened flavored water
FUZE slenderize Tropical Punch beverage
Heavenly Desserts™ Sugar Free Fat Free Meringue*
   Lemon, cappuccino, chocolate, strawberry and vanilla
1 bottle Kiwi, Berry or Orange Propel-Free

Ordering information in appendix

Eating Out

The moment has hit and you're ready to take your show on the road. Perhaps you were forced to skip a home-cooked meal due to a business meeting, kid's soccer game, or a long day at work. This means you need to put on your portion-size hat and get familiar with the dining-out guidelines for The Tropical Diet program.

This is not an unusual situation. In fact, most of you eat out 50% more than a few decades ago, 200% more at fast foods restaurants alone. Even snacking has increased 50%.

The problem is not with eating out but with the portion sizes. Research shows that the portion sizes of restaurant foods have actually grown six-fold in the last two decades at most major restaurant chains. For instance, a soda 20 years ago was approximately 6.5 ounces and 85 calories. Today your soda is super-sized at 20 ounces, and typically has 250 calories, 100% sugar. Another example is your standard turkey sandwich. Twenty years ago it had about 320 calories while today that same sandwich has typically grown to 820 calories. What's more startling is the large portion sizes have carried over to our home cooking.

And these larger portion sizes have also gotten back to your cookbooks. Take for instance, *The Joy of Cooking's* brownie recipe. In 1975, it yielded 30 servings. Today the same recipe yields 16. Another cookbook example is the 1984 recipe for Toll House cookies which yielded 100 servings. Today it only yields 60.

That can really hurt your efforts to lose weight. What is a Tropical Dieter to do? Know your portion sizes, food options, and get a sense of the best choices at all your favorite ethnic or fast food restaurants.

By all means, there is no way all your options will be presented in this section. And fast food places are updating their healthier food choices as we speak. So, if you have a question about eating out, about the food or recipe selections, email *www.thetropicaldiet.com* website, ask your Tropical Diet nutritionist or a registered dietitian for advice about eating out. You can also log onto many of the fast food restaurant websites by name and they will provide the actual nutritional analysis of your meal and show you optional analyses for healthier options.

IN THE BEGINNING

Starting your day on the wrong foot can also add hundreds of unnecessary fat and carbohydrate calories. For instance, the ordinary plain frozen Lender's bagel has 160 calories, the equivalent of two slices of bread. However if you plan to venture out to your local bagel shop, this is what you might find:

Morning Breakfast Chart

Restaurant Dunkin Donuts	Calories	Fat (grams)	Equivalent to "" slices of bread
Plain bagel	210	1	"2¾"
Cinnamon raisin	230	2	"3"
Au Bon Pain			
Plain	380	2	"4¾"
Cinnamon	395	2	"5"
Sesame	425	5 (one fat serving)	"5½"
Add two tablespoons of: Cream cheese			You get an additional: 99 calories and 10 grams fat

In the case of the bagel, here's my advice. Buy yourself a bag of Lender's bagels and store them in the fridge. Invite your friend over for some fresh fruit, coffee, and a toasted bagel with fat-free toppings.

If you choose to meet your friend for breakfast, just have ½ of a plain bagel with non-fat cream cheese, or jelly. You can also order it toasted topped with lettuce, and tomato for an extra fiber boost. Still hungry? Get a side of fresh fruit salad, and finish breakfast off with a soothing cup of coffee prepared with low-fat milk.

You can have all that and you'll save:

Before	Calories	Tropical Diet™ Breakfast Makeover	Calories
1 Au Bon Pain cinnamon bagel	598	½ plain bagel	190 cal
With cream cheese and jelly		toasted with tomato and lettuce	10 cal
Coffee with cream	50	Coffee with nonfat milk	20 cal
		Fruit salad cup	100 cal
Total Calories and fat:	**648/22grams**		**320/2 grams**

Total Savings with Tropical Diet Breakfast:
328 calories and 20 grams fat (180 calories fat)

Now you can see how critical it can be to take charge of your dining-out experiences so you don't skip a beat with your program even while maintaining an active social life.

Here are some additional guidelines you can follow:

1. Know your portion sizes.

As I showed you, you can't rely on portion sizes. For instance, one Tropical Diet starch portion of bread is approx 80 calories (1 oz.). In the real world, you're served a portion with 3.7 oz. and almost 400 calories. A 1/2 cup Tropical Diet fruit serving of juice is 60 calories. In the real world, you get 1½ cups and 180 calories.

Here are some other examples:

TD Food portions	In the Real World
½ cup cooked veggies, 25 calories	1½ cups with butter, 120 calories
2-3 protein oz. servings lean meat, 240 cal	12 oz. steak, 960 calories
1 oz. lite or fat free salad dressing,10 to 30 cal	3 oz. high fat dressing, 270 calories

So the key is to have your Tropical Diet portion size cheat sheet with you at all times when eating out until you get the hang of your *L.A.B.* plan serving guide and amounts. This will help you manage your calorie intake and stay on track.

2. Don't be shy. Get foods made to order.

Find out the ingredients in your foods if you are unsure of the preparation. Don't assume that grilled means without a brush of oil. Ask for salads with dressing on the side, main courses with sauces on the side.

3. Be creative.

Order an assortment of appetizers like soup and shrimp cocktail or side dishes like baked potato and steamed veggies if these foods meet your diet guidelines more accurately than the main dishes.

4. Don't give in.

Stick to your game plan—stop eating at the places that sabotage your diet efforts and try new ones.

5. Become ethnically food savvy.

Learn what to order at your favorite Chinese, Japanese, Greek, Italian, Mexican, Thai, or other ethnic restaurants. Here are some broad guidelines you can follow.

The Tropical Diet Ethnic Eating-Out Guide

CHINESE

Chinese cuisine actually reflects a variety of cuisines from various regions including Canton, Hunan, Mandarin, Peking (Beijing) or Shanghai, or Szechwan. Each region has its own menu style which would be too lengthy to describe for this guide, however here are some of your best Chinese food choices overall:

Order This:	Instead of This:
Clear soups like wonton, hot and sour, Vegetable or steamed wonton or potsticker appetizers	fried appetizers like egg rolls, and wontons
Braised, simmered, roasted and steamed Vegetable, fish or white meat chicken, Chow mein dishes loaded with veggies, minus the MSG	stir-fried dishes, fried rice items, sweet 'n sour anything!

CHINESE (cont'd)

Order This:	Instead of This:
Wonton cookie	ice cream, fried noodles, almond cookies, frozen or sweet drinks.

When available, order hot or Szechwan for a metabolic boost!

FRENCH

Order This:	Instead of This:
Clear consommés	cream soup
Demiglace sauces	cheese, creamy sauces
Roasted or braised meat, poultry or fish	croissants
Salads, steamed veggies	French fries, rich desserts

ITALIAN

Order This:	Instead of This:
Thin crust pizza with veggies and without cheese *(Sprinkle some parmesan on for the cheese effect!)*	deep crusted cheesy, pepperoni, anchovies, bacon, extra cheese, prosciutto, sausage
Italian bread	garlic rolls, parmesan bread, or bruschetta.
Minestrone or vegetable soup	cream soup
Salads with dressing on the side	antipasto
Pasta with red sauce	pasta with cream or cheese sauce
Italian fruit or ice	cannoli pastries

JAPANESE:

Order This:	Instead of This:
Oshitashi appetizer—*spinach/asparagus*	spring rolls, fried tofu,
Vegetable, shrimp or crab sushi	tuna, eel, or salmon sushi
Low sodium soy sauce, wasabi, ginger	regular soy sauce
Clear vegetable or miso soup	tempura appetizers or main course

JAPANESE: (cont'd)

Order This: **Instead of This:**

Salad with dressing on the side

Simmered or grilled dishes   breaded and fried dishes like tonkatsu

Udon or soba soups   fried vegetarian main courses

Fresh fruit or sorbet   fried ice cream

Green iced or hot tea for an antioxidant lift

MEXICAN

Order This: **Instead of This:**

Salad and black bean soup   nachos, potato skins or refried bean dip
                                                   any salad or soup with sour cream

Fresh corn tortilla   flour or fried tortilla

Fajita, soft tacos, burritos minus the cheese   grande, double and combo dishes loaded with cheese

Side of black beans and rice   refried beans with cheese and rice

Fruit or sherbet dessert   fried ice cream

INDIAN

Order This: **Instead of This:**

Lentil or mulligatawny soup   fried appetizers

Vegetable curry   fried vegetable dishes

Side dishes with veggies beans or peas   fried breads like chapatti, nan, roti

Tandoori chicken or tikka   dishes with coconut milk

Biryani-rice dish with veggies, fruits,   anything with ghee (clarified butter)
nuts or meat

THAI

Order This: **Instead of This:**

Broth based soup tom yum koong   soups with coconut milk

THAI (cont'd)

Order This:	Instead of This:
Thai salad with dressing on the side	fried appetizers that say crispy
Basil, chili or ginger dishes for the love boost!	Anything made with coconut milk
Steamed veggies, steamed rice	fried veggies or rice
Grilled meats, chicken, fish	fried banana or desserts prepared with coconut milk

Make It Fast

Fast food restaurants have been hit the hardest lately by the government and the press as one of the leading causes of obesity in this country. Larger portion sizes, a 200% increase in fast food dining over the past two decades, and economics may be three of the main reasons for the blame. In response, the fast food industry has developed healthier food items, all that fit into your Tropical Diet plan.

Here is the list of the best fast food choices that you can include on your *Convenience Cuisine©* menus when you're running out of time, ingredients, or are just "on-the-run".

*Fast Food Best Bets for Convenience Cuisine© Menu Planning**

Arbys
Sourdough with ham for breakfast
Caesar salad without dressing
Caesar side salad

Burger King
Veggie burger, no mayo
Garden salad, lite or nonfat dressing
Chicken Caesar salad, lite or fat-free
    dressing

Jamba Juice—*under 300 calories*
Caribbean Passion® (sixteen)
Cranberry Craze® (sixteen)
Orange Berry Blitz™ (sixteen)
Orange-A-Peel™ (sixteen)
Orange-Carrot (sixteen or original)
Protein Berry Pizzazz™ (sixteen)
Vibrant-C® (sixteen)

McDonald's
Chicken McGrill, no mayo
Regular hamburger with lettuce,
tomato, mustard & ketchup
Yogurt cup
English muffin, plain
Orange juice, lowfat milk, or water

Pizza Hut
1 slice personal pan, *Veggie Lover's,*
or *Quartered Ham*
1 slice *Chicken Supreme*
1 slice Fit 'n Delicious
2 hot chicken wings
salad with lite dressing

Quiznos
Small Sierra Smoked Turkey
Small Honey Bourbon Chicken
Small Turkey Lite®
Salads, lite or fat-free dressing, no olives
cheese or bacon

Smoothie King—*under 15 calories per oz.*
Caribbean Way®
GoGuava™
Slim & Trim™ Vanilla and Orange-
Vanilla

Subway
Whole-wheat bread for:
6" Veggie Delite®
Roast beef, ham, chicken breast, or
turkey—no cheese, no mayo
Veggie, chicken breast, turkey
Roast beef or club salad—fat-free
Italian or red wine vinaigrette
Mediterranean chicken Atkins® friendly
salad
Vegetarian vegetable soup

Taco Bell
Plain taco
Soft taco chicken or grilled steak
Gordita Baja® steak or chicken
Echinito® steak

Wendys
Garden Sensation™ Salads
Mandarin Chicken salad
Spring Mix Salad
Side or Caesar side salad
Small chili
Lite salad dressing
Baked potato—plain
Jr. Hamburger
Junior Frosty®

---

*choices based on assessment of nutrient analysis provided by company website information.

ℒ.𝒜.ℬ. Menus and Recipes

The menus for The Tropical Diet program are designed for flexibility—regardless of your lifestyle, desires, and tastes, you will find the dishes, beverages, and snacks you like to consume are accessible and affordable to you. The menus are located in your ℒ.𝒜.ℬ. plan chapters: Chapter 5-ℒean, Chapter 6 𝒜thlete, and Chapter 7—ℬasic.

The food, fluid, and snacking recommendations are designed to help you meet all your essential needs for protein, carbohydrates, fats, vitamins, minerals, phytochemicals, and fiber for health, sport, and life. Some food and fluid choices are included just for fun and pleasure—remember the comfort foods from your Food Fitness, and Pleasure Pyramid in Chapter 2. If you are unfamiliar with a tropical food item, just jump over to the Glossary and look it up. They're in alphabetical order. Recipes are located at the end of this chapter beginning on page 170.

While this book offers you a variety of drink, appetizer, soup, salad, chicken, fish, pork, and dessert recipes, it is by no means a comprehensive guide to cooking, nor a complete and authentic Caribbean cookbook. It merely provides you with a taste of tropical cuisine so you become tempted to purchase the other fabulous cookbooks listed in the Appendix. In the meantime, plans are already underway for a *Tropical Diet Cookbook*—recipes, cooking lessons, and a CD-ROM to teach you how to prepare Tropical Diet™ foods from scratch.

How to Use the Menus

By selecting a variety of food choices for each day, you can conceivably eat something nutritious and different for several weeks before getting bored with the program. You can also play it safe and stick to the same foods and rotate them on a weekly basis. Either way, you can be assured of a healthy diet.

For instance, if the breakfast menu calls for scrambled egg whites, fruit juice, and toast, you can change over to low-fat cottage cheese with fresh pineapple and berries the next day, or have an energy bar and coffee the following day with a midmorning snack of cheese and apple. Remember, you can always make the switch (see Chapter 3) to another plan if you get bored, hit a plateau, or need a break.

GOURMET, CONVENIENCE, OR FAST FOOD CUISINE

You'll find three menu options, *Tropical Diet Gourmet Cuisine, Convenience Cuisine©* or *Fast Food Cuisine.*

If you're the type who likes to take the time to prepare, and eat fresh, home-cooked meals, you will enjoy The *Tropical Diet Gourmet Cuisine* menu option. Many of these recipe items have been developed by the book's chef expert, Michelle Austin and adapted from the Tropical Diet Spa Cuisine program launched at some of the Caribbean's finest resorts. You will also be able to prepare some of the recipes from the upcoming *Krome Avenue Cookbook*, available at The Fruit and Spice Park in Homestead, Florida.

For busy dieters with less time to spend on home prepared meals, The Tropical Diet *Convenience Cuisine©* menu items are for you. These choices provide a combination of homemade foods which can be prepared in advance in bulk quantities, and refrigerated, or frozen for later use. About 50 to 75% of the items are fresh, natural, and homemade. *Convenience Cuisine©* food choices, quick beverages, bars, or fast food cuisines make up the bulk of the menu items. The *Convenience Cuisine©* will still ensure the nutritional value of your diet while helping you save time and lose weight whether you're a full-time professional, homemaker, or frequent traveler.

If you feel you might fall into The *Tropical Fast Food Junkie* category, mostly eating on the run if you stop to eat at all, you can have your cake and eat it, too. The goal of these menu selections is to introduce healthy foods to the fast food eater's diet, to enhance their present diets with tropical food, or beverage ingredients, and to do this with the least amount of work, worry, or preparation.

Most of the fast food restaurants offer healthier selections, and will continue to improve their menus since they have taken the brunt of most of the obesity epidemic blame from the government, the public, and the press. You will be able to eat-on-the-fly and stay on your program as long as you enhance the quality of your meals with additional vegetable, fruit, and whole-grain servings, low-fat dairy, sport drinks, and bars, and minimize the amount of fat, saturated fat, cholesterol, and sodium you consume from fast food meals. These menus provide 0 to 50% fresh, natural, and homemade foods. Other food choices include name-brand or convenience foods which happen to be tropically flavored or enhanced ready-to-eat meals, snacks, shakes or energy bars meals. At a minimum, the fast food tropical cuisine will be:

- Portion-controlled.
- Will introduce healthy foods into a less-than-perfect eating regimen.
- Will nutritionally enhance the diet regardless of its present state.

Be sure to balance any plan with daily exercise, adequate fluids and relaxation techniques and regardless of how much time you spend in the kitchen, you too will be a healthy Tropical Dieter.

Special Appearances

Throughout this chapter's menus, recipes, and nutrient analysis sections, you will find valuable bits and pieces of food, fitness, and culinary tidbits, which I have highlighted in a variety of ways to make them easy to spot.

These nutritional sidebars will look like this:

◉ *Nutrition Nugget*

These provide cool and cutting-edge information about the food, vitamin, and mineral content or overall health issues relating to the topic addressed.

Chef Michelle's Tips

These include Chef Michelle's advice for preparation, cooking techniques, seasoning, and substitutions.

📖 CHRIS NOTES:

These are practical suggestions, personal observations, and professional tips from Chris Rollins, international tropical food expert and director of the Fruit and Spice Park, Homestead, Florida.

The Best Five Ways to
Tropically Dress-Up Your Menus

Regardless of whether you choose the spa, convenience, or fast food cuisine, there are specific ways you can boost the nutritional quality of your meals simply by including a tropical food, fruit, vegetable, or spice. Additional healthy recommendations are included throughout the book in the |⚫| Nutrition Nuggets.

1. Season your food with nutritious seasonings such as basil, mint, and ginger or any of the nutritious seasonings listed in the chart on page 154.
2. Drink one cup of orange, grapefruit, cranberry, or grape juice with meat, bean, and whole grain dishes to help absorb additional iron and add valuable antioxidants to your meal.
3. Keep a bag of frozen or canned low-sodium, mixed vegetables in your refrigerator, and add a cup to your lunch and dinner meals to salads, soups, and side dishes.
4. Achieve the *fabulous five,* 5 colors at every meal by adding:

   • Orange—papaya, mango, cantaloupe, or carrots.
   • Green—kiwi, leafy vegetables, peas, or broccoli.
   • White—non-fat milk or dairy products.
   • Brown—whole grains, beans, or meats.
   • Red—tomatoes, strawberries, or watermelon.

5. Eat a serving of fish, soy, or ground flaxseed to add essential omega-3 fats for healthy blood pressure and healing and a beautiful mind.

Medicinal and Nutritive Seasoning Chart

HERB	MEDICINAL	NUTRIEINTS
Dill	Diuretic, may aid digestion	Potassium, calcium, magnesium
Anise	Diuretic, stimulant, eliminates gas	Potassium, calcium, phosphorus
Bay Leaf	Antiseptic, digestive aid	Vitamin A, potassium, and calcium
Oregano	Antiseptic, facilitates digestion, eases migraines, and motion sickness	Calcium, potassium, magnesium, vitamin A
Basil	Antiseptic tonic, fights migraine, digestive aid, insomniac remedy	Potassium, calcium,phosphorus, magnesium, vitamin A
Thyme	Diuretic, stimulates perspiration and relieves gas	Calcium, potassium, iron, magnesium, phosphorus and vitamin A
Parsley	Breath freshener, stimulant	Vitamin A, C, phosphorus, potassium, and calcium
Mint	Antiseptic, aphrodisiac, stimulant	Calcium, potassium, magnesium
Rosemary	Diuretic, stimulant, gas reliever, stimulates perspiration	Calcium, potassium, magnesium
Saffron	Digestive, gas reliever	Potassium and phosphorus
Cumin	Antiseptic, stimulant	Calcium and potassium
Ginger	Diuretic, antiseptic, digestive aid, combats gas, pain	Potassium, magnesium and phosphorus

HERB	MEDICINAL	NUTRIEINTS
Black Pepper	Antibacterial, stimulants and aids digestion	Potassium, calcium, phosphorus and magnesium
Chili Pepper	Metabolic booster, to eliminate burning in mouth, eat yogurt, bread, cooked rice, sugar, and sweets	Vitamins A and C

*Nutritional Analysis of Recipes, Menus and L.A.B. plans**

The Tropical Diet menus, *L.A.B.* profiles, and recipes were analyzed using the ESHA Food Processor SQL computerized nutritional analysis program. The nutrient information in the ESHA databases is compiled from over 1,300 scientific sources. The program takes the latest United States Department of Agriculture (USDA) data and then adds additional foods, ingredients, and brand-name products researched from manufacturers.

The extra efforts ESHA takes to ensure the nutritional accuracy of the data is:

- Data from scientific journal articles are used to fill in the many missing values for important trace vitamins and minerals and other nutrient factors.
- When there are several sources for a nutrient in a food item, they combine data with regard to the number of analyses used to report a value and then weigh values accordingly.
- Where appropriate, data is imputed from similar food items to minimize missing values. Errors and missing values are further minimized with quality-control reviews.

Nutrients analyzed for each item include over 165 nutrients, including vitamins, minerals, amino acids (proteins), saturated fatty acids, monounsaturated fatty acids, polyunsaturated fatty acids, trans fatty acids, dietary fiber fractions, sugar, organic acids, sugar alcohols, and others.

Compu-Cal hand-held calculator and dietary analysis program was utilized to calculate the *L.A.B.* program's analysis for every calorie level, protein, carbohydrates, and fats according to the ADA dietary exchange program.

———————

*Adapted from ESHA Company manual and website *www.esha.com.*

The Tropical Diet

ᴌᴇᴀɴ Pʀᴏɢʀᴀᴍ Mᴇɴᴜ ᴀɴᴅ Sɴᴀᴄᴋ Cʜᴏɪᴄᴇs

On the ᴌean program, the best way to think of your daily meal choices is to imagine a handful of protein-rich foods, about 4 to 6 oz. at each meal—eggs, fish, non-fat cheese, chicken, turkey, lean meats, and pork, served with generous portions of colorful vegetables, a few slices of tropical fruit, and pinch of fat from oil, nuts, or additional fats contributed from the cooking process.

Beverage Choices

Hot water with lemon

Sparkling water with lemon or key lime

Propel Water-kiwi strawberry or any fruit flavor

Green tea

Peppermint iced tea

Chamomile tea

Trop Coco™ Coconut Water

FUZE Slenderize Drink

Fruit flavored seltzers

Coffee

Coffee beverages without sugar

Special Occasions—Key Lime Vodka Martini (1 fruit, 1 fat)

Glass wine—(2 fruits)

EAS™ AdvantEdge® Drink (contributes 2 protein servings)

On the Light Side

A quick snack or lite bite before your main course.

Fresh and Natural	Gourmet Cuisine	Convenience Cuisine©
Pineapple with mint	Island Vegetable Tian*	Low-carb breakfast bars
Kiwi slices	Ceviche Key Lime Shot*	PowerBar® ProteinPlus™ Bar
Papaya with lime	Tuna Tartar on Plantain	String Cheese
Guava with mint	Wafer*	Small box raisins
Watermelon with mint		A "shotful" of soy nuts
Mango with mint		EAS™ AdvantEdge® Drink

Orange slices
Grapefruit sections
Berries with nonfat yogurt dip
Jicama sticks with guacamole
Baby carrots with lowfat ranch dressing
Radishes with lowfat dip

Soup

Something warm to soothe your spirit and calm your hunger pangs.

Fresh and Natural	Gourmet Cuisine	Convenience Cuisine©
Any clear consommé	Brocco Consommé*	Miso soup
Lite and clear vegetable soup	Chicken soup	

Salad

Crunchy, fresh, and lite for any meal, any time of day.

Fresh and Natural	Gourmet Cuisine	Convenience Cuisine©
Tossed salad	Chayote Salad Slaw*	Wendy's Salad
Spinach salad	Crab, Ginger, and Grapefruit	Sensations
Bagged salad from grocery	Salad*	McDonald's Salad
Coleslaw	Mango Strawberry and	shaker or grilled
	Christophene Salad	chicken salad
		Subway turkey, club
		or ham salad
		Burger King side salad or broiled
		Chicken Salad
		Arby's Roast Chicken Salad
		Taco Bell lowfat salads

Main Course
The heart of the meal.

Fresh and Natural	Gourmet Cuisine	Convenience Cuisine©
Egg white omelette	Cinnamon Tuna Steak*	Fast-food salads as
Steak, pan fried with Pam	Jerk Kingfish*	main course
(Omaha®, 4 oz. flat steaks)	Island Pork*	Atkins Friendly® wraps
Chicken breast, grilled or	Shrimp & Vegetable Skewer*	Healthy Choice™ Meal
pan fried with Pam	Mahi Mahi Tropical*	
Sliced turkey with greens	Caribbean Ginger Chicken*	
	Vegetable Lasagna*	

Dessert

fruit or combination of fruit	Baked Quince*	Fat-free, sugar-free
on kabob with yogurt dip	Lychees with Strawberry	Popsicle
	Dressing*	Frozen berries with
	Key Lime Vodka Martini	Nonfat whipped cream
		Sugar-free, fat-free meringue
		Sugar-free, fat-free hot chocolate

—————————

*Tropical Diet recipes on pages 170-221

⊿EAN PLAN SNACK CHOICES

Snacking is a great way to tropically spruce up your menus, and include the healthy ingredients necessary for a nutritious diet.

Free Snack Choices
Green leafy salad with oil-free vinaigrette
FUZE™ Tropical Punch Slenderize Drink
Propel flavored water
Fruit flavored seltzers
Fresh Radishes
Green tea
Brewed decaf and regular coffee

Snacks **under 50 calories to 75 calories**
Trop Coco™ coconut water
1 orange, apple or pear, sliced
24 grapes

Snacks under 50 calories to 75 calories (cont'd)
10 fresh Lychee
1 kiwi, carambola, grapefruit, or prickly pear
½ c. fresh pineapple,
1 c. papaya, strawberries or watermelon
1 guava
1 baked quince
1 cup raw celery, jicama and red pepper with 1 oz. fat-free dressing
Bristol Meyers® Squib Choice Berry Almond Crisp Bar
Guilt Free™ sugar-free, fat free fudge bar
Dole® papaya in peach gelatin
1 c. Tropicana® Light and Healthy Orange Juice
Stretch Island® Truly Tropical or Mucho Mango Fruit Leather
Kettle Valley® Tropical Blend Fruit Snack
Brisol-Meyers® Squib Choice Fiber Bursts, tropical fruit flavor *

Snacks under 100 calories
11 almonds
7 walnuts
1 lowfat string cheese
½ c. frozen jackfruit
1 small frozen banana
2 oz. tofu
2 oz. Lifeline® fat-free cheese
Cottage cheese, *fat-free,* with 1 oz. blueberries
Yoplait® *fat-free* Strawberry Banana yogurt
Bristol Meyers® Squib Diabetic Choice™ Drink, vanilla or strawberry
10 Gold Mine organic mungbean chips
EAS™ AdvantEdge® low-carb drink
Primal Spirit® Foods Primal Soy Strips
½ c. Woodstock Farms® tropical fruit mix
17 Carbo LITE™ gummy bears

Snacks under 150 calories
1 mango, black sapote, sapodilla or pomegranate
1 oz. soy nuts
¼ c. Woodstock Farms® Cascade trail mix

Snacks under 200 calories

PowerBar® ProteinPlus™ sugar-free apple caramel bar
1 c. Stonyfield® fat-free vanilla yogurt
EAS™ Myoplex Carb Sense Drink

---

* Sugar-free, fiber supplement with 3 grams dietary fiber

ᴀTHLETE PLAN MENU AND SNACK CHOICES

On the ᴀthlete's plan, you'll find all the same foods and menu suggestions from the ᴌean plan however, additional portions of carbohydrate-based foods like pastas, rice, couscous, potatoes, and grains are also included. Visualize your plate with a handful of chicken, fish, or meat with fruits, vegetables, and sport drinks, sport bars, gels, and beverages to fuel the active Tropical Dieter.

Beverages

Fresh and Natural	Gourmet Cuisine	Convenience Cuisine©
Fruit smoothies	Ginger-Papaya Cocktail*	Smoothie-King®
Hot water with lemon	Mango Madness Cocktail*	smoothies
Sparkling water with lemon or	Pomegranate Morning Cocktail*	Jamba Juice®
Key lime	*Special Occasions*—Key Lime Vodka	smoothies
Propel Water—kiwi strawberry	Martini (1 fruit, 1 fat)	Starbucks®
or any fruit flavor	1 glass wine (2 fruits)	drinks with
Green tea	1 beer (2 starches)	non or low
Peppermint iced tea		fat milk
Chamomile tea		
Trop Coco™ Coconut Water		
FUZE™ Slenderize		
Fruit flavored seltzers		
Brewed coffee		
Coffee beverages without sugar		
Café con leche, café Cubano		
EAS™ AdvantEdge® Drink		
(Contributes 2 protein servings)		
EAS™ Myoplex™ Carb Sense Drink		
(3 protein, ½ fat)		

On The Light Side

A quick snack or lite bite before your main course.

Fresh and Natural	Gourmet Cuisine	Convenience Cuisine©
Pineapple with mint	Island Vegetable Tian*	Apple, pear or orange
Cantaloupe with mint	Ceviche Key Lime Shot*	PowerBar® ProteinPlus™ Bar
Papaya with lime	Tuna Tartar on Plantain	Banana
Guava with mint	Wafer*	Small box raisins
Watermelon with mint	Vegetable Crudités	EAS™ AdvantEdge® Drink
Kiwi slices	with lima bean dip*	A shotful of Tropical
Mango with mint	Baked tortilla chips	Trail Mix
Orange slices	with avocado or fruit salsa	
Grapefruit sections		
Berries with nonfat yogurt dip		
Jicama sticks with guacamole		
Baby carrots with low fat ranch dressing		
Radishes with low fat dip		

Soup

Something warm to soothe your spirit and calm your hunger pangs.

Fresh and Natural	Gourmet Cuisine	Convenience Cuisine©
Any clear consommé	Brocco Consommé*	Miso soup*
Lite and clear vegetable Soup	Miami Style Black	Chicken soup*
	Bean Soup*	Minestrone soup*
	Gingered Carrot and Pear	Chicken noodle soup*
	Bisque*	*low sodium soups
	Island Vegetable Soup*	
	Vegetarian Chili*	

Salad

Crunchy, fresh, and lite for any meal, any time of day.

Fresh and Natural	Gourmet Cuisine	Convenience Cuisine©
Tossed salad	Chayote Salad Slaw*	Wendy's Salad
Spinach salad	Crab, Ginger, and Grapefruit	Sensations
Carrot-raisin salad	Salad*	McDonald's Salad
Coleslaw	Mango Strawberry and	Shaker or grilled
	Christophene Salad*	chicken salad
	Chayote, Corn, and Chili	Subway's turkey, club
	Toss*	or ham salad
		Burger King side salad or
		broiled chicken salad

Salad (cont'd)

Fresh and Natural	Gourmet Cuisine	Convenience Cuisine©
		Arby's Roast Chicken Salad
		Taco Bell lowfat salads
		Subway 6" Sub on whole wheat, no mayo

Main Course

The heart of the meal.

Fresh and Natural	Gourmet Cuisine	Convenience Cuisine©
Whole grain cereal/oats with nonfat milk	Tropical Fruit Pancakes* with fruit sauce*	Vegetable sushi or hand roll
Egg white omelette	Cinnamon Tuna Steak*	Fast food salads as main course
Steak—pan fried with Pam (Omaha 4 oz. flat steaks)	Jerk Kingfish*	
	Island Pork*	Atkins Friendly wraps
Chicken breast, grilled or pan fried with Pam	Shrimp and Vegetable Skewer*	Healthy Choice™ Meals
	Mahi Mahi Tropical*	
Sliced turkey roll in pasta with red sauce	Caribbean Ginger Chicken*	
	Vegetable Lasagna*	
Steamed vegetables with baked potato	Tropical Mougrabiya*	
	Spaghetti squash with red sauce*	
	Pasta Tropical*	
	Christophene Gratin*	
	Carrot and Pumpkin Risotto*	
	Boiled Plantains*	
	Black beans with Tomato and Bell Pepper*	
	Chicken Wrap*	

Dessert

Fresh and Natural	Gourmet Cuisine	Convenience Cuisine©
Any fruit or combination of fruits from appetizer list in bowl, on kabob with yogurt dip, or frozen with fat-free whipped cream sugar-free, fat-free frozen	Baked Quince*	TCBY,™ or any lowfat frozen yogurt
	Lychees with Strawberry Dressing*	Italian ices
	Key Lime Vodka Martini*	sorbet
	Baked Goods:	meringue
	Gingered Papaya Muffins*	

Dessert (cont'd)

Fresh and Natural	Gourmet Cuisine	Convenience Cuisine©
fruit pops	Confetti Cornbread*	
Sugar-free, fat-free meringue	Garbanzo Cake*	
Sugar-free, fat-free hot chocolate	Papaya Jack Coffee Cake*	
with non-fat whipped cream	Tropical Tres Leche*	
	Rose Flan*	
	Tropical Brownies*	

*A*THLETE PLAN

Snack Choices
Free Snack Choices
Green leafy salad with oil free vinaigrette
FUZE™ Tropical Punch Slenderize Drink-Sugar Free
Propel flavored water
Syfo fruit flavored seltzers
Fresh radishes
Green tea
Brewed decaf and regular coffee

Snacks under 50 calories to 75 calories
1 orange, apple or pear slices
24 grapes
10 fresh lychee
1 kiwi, carambola, grapefruit, prickly pear
½ c. fresh pineapple,
1 c. papaya, strawberries or watermelon
1 guava
1 baked quince
1 cup raw celery, jicama and red pepper with fat-free dip
Bristol Meyers Squib Choice Berry Almond Crisp Bar
Guilt Free™ Fudge Bar
Dole® Papaya in Peach Gel
1 c. Tropicana® Light and Healthy Orange Juice
Stretch Island Truly Tropical or Mucho Mango fruit leather
Kettle Valley Tropical Blend fruit snack
3 Soken® seaweed candies
3 Brisol-Meyers Squib Tropical Fruit Choice Fiber Burst*

Snacks under 100 calories

11 almonds

7 walnuts

2 fresh figs

1 low fat string cheese

½ c. frozen jackfruit

1 frozen small banana

2 oz. Caribbean Tofu

cottage cheese, fat free with blueberries

Yoplait fat-free Strawberry Banana yogurt

Bristol Meyers Squib Diabetic Choice Vanilla or Strawberry Drink

4 c. air blown popcorn

20 Pennysticks oat bran pretzel nuggets

10 Gold Mine organic mungbean chips

12 baked tortilla chips

EAS™ AdvantEdge® drink

Primal Spirit® Foods Primal Soy Strips

Del Monte Mandarin oranges

25 GeniSoy® Salt 'n Vinegar Soy Crisps

¼ c. Woodstock Farms tropical fruit mix

17 Carbo LITE gummy bears

Miss Meringue™ classic meringue cookies

1 Jogmate™

Snacks under 150 calories

1 mango, black sapote, sapodilla or pomegranate

⅓ c. Tropical hi energy trail mix

Vruit™ tropical blend juice pack

Nutribiotic apple strawberry bar

Dannon Light èn Fit smoothie

Diabetic Care, Choice Chocolate Fudge Drink

4 c. Bearitos air blown popcorn—no salt/oil flavored

1 Fruitfull® Strawberry Cream or banana frozen fruit bar

1 oz. soy nuts

1 bag Hot Mate Assorted Rice Cracker Snax

8 Valley Lahvosh heart crackers

¼ c. Woodstock Farms Cascade Trail Mix

1 scoop Accelerade® sport drink

Aunt Gussie's fat-free, sugar-free orange biscottini

1 Tropical flavor Power gel®

Snacks under 200 calories

PowerBar® ProteinPlus™ sugar-free apple caramel bar

1 c. Stonyfield® fat-free vanilla yogurt

1 bag Glenny's® Cheddar Soy crisps

GeniSoy® Extreme Crunch Island blast bar

Myoplex™ Carb Sense French Vanilla Drink

1 bag Glenny's® salt n pepper or lightly salted soy crisps

1 c. West Soy® Tropical Whip Smoothie

Sharkies® Berry Blast Organic Energy Fruit Chews

Luna® Bar Tropical Crisp Bar

9 Kasugai Kiwi or Muscat Gummy Candies

---

* Sugar free, fiber supplement with 3 grams dietary fiber

ℬASIC PLAN MENUS

The ℬasic Plan menus differ from the ℒean and 𝒜thlete Plan menus, because there is a greater emphasis on the even distribution of protein, fat, and carbohydrates at each meal and snack. And while all the ℒean Plan choices work on these menus, the high-carbohydrate 𝒜thlete Plan choices do not. High glycemic index (page 100) carbohydrates are not recommended. Many of the starch-based entrees from the 𝒜thlete plan are not suitable for this program. Think of your plate divided into three portions with a greater emphasis on the protein, a thumbnail or two of oil or fat, a healthy portion of colorful vegetables, and a small helping of sliced tropical fruits.

Beverage Choices

Hot water with lemon
Sparkling water with lemon or key lime
Propel® Water-kiwi strawberry or any fruit flavor
Green tea
Peppermint iced tea
Chamomile tea
Trop Coco™ Coconut Water
FUZE Slenderize
Fruit-flavored seltzers
Coffee
Coffee beverages without sugar
Special Occasions—Key Lime Vodka Martini (1 fruit, 1 fat)
Glass wine—(2 fruits)
EAS™ AdvantEdge® Drink (contributes 2 protein servings)

On the Light Side

A quick snack or lite bite before your main course.

Fresh and Natural	Gourmet Cuisine	Convenience Cuisine©
Pineapple with mint	Island Vegetable Tian*	PowerBar® ProteinPlus™ Bar
Cantaloupe with mint	Ceviche Shot*	1 banana
Papaya with lime	Tuna Tartar on Plantain	EAS™ AdvantEdge® Bar
Guava with mint	wafer*	EAS™ AdvantEdge® Drink
Watermelon with mint		1 shotful of soy nuts or
Kiwi slices		trail mix
Mango with mint		LifeLine fat-free
Orange slices		cheese with apple slices
Grapefruit sections		
Berries with low fat yogurt dip		
Jicama sticks with guacamole		
Baby carrots with low fat ranch dressing		
Radishes with low fat dip		

Soup

Something warm to soothe your spirit and calm your hunger pangs.

Fresh and Natural	Gourmet Cuisine	Convenience Cuisine©
Any clear consommé	Brocco Consommé*	miso soup
Lite and clear vegetable Soup		chicken soup

Salad

Crunchy fresh and lite for any meal, any time of day.

Fresh and Natural	Gourmet Cuisine	Convenience Cuisine©
Tossed salad	Chayote Salad Slaw*	Wendy's Salad
Spinach salad	Crab, Ginger, and Grapefruit	Sensations
Bagged salad from grocery	Salad*	McDonald's Salad
Coleslaw	Mango, Strawberry and	Shaker or grilled
	Christophene Salad*	Chicken salad
		Subway turkey, club
		or ham salad
		Burger King side salad
		or broiled
		Chicken Salad
		Arby's roast chicken
		salad
		Taco Bell low fat salads

Main Course

The heart of the meal.

Fresh and Natural	Gourmet Cuisine	Convenience Cuisine©
Egg white omelette	Cinnamon Tuna Steak*	Fast food salads as main
Steak—pan fried with Pam	Jerk Kingfish*	course
(Omaha® 4 oz. flat steaks)	Island Pork*	Atkins Friendly wraps
Chicken breast, grilled or	Shrimp and Vegetable Skewer*	Healthy Choice™ Meals
pan fried with Pam	Mahi Mahi Tropical*	
	Caribbean Ginger Chicken*	
	Cured Tuna Scented with	
	Coriander, Brunoise of	
	Vegetables*	

Desserts

Fresh and Natural	Gourmet Cuisine	Convenience Cuisine©
Any fruit or combination of fruits from appetizer list in bowl, on kabob with yogurt dip, or frozen with fat free whipped cream sugar-free, fat-free frozen fruit pops Sugar-free, fat-free meringue Sugar-free, fat-free hot chocolate with non-fat whipped cream	Baked Quince* Lychees with Strawberry Dressing* Key Lime Vodka Martini	TCBY® sugar free yogurt Trail mix Energy bars

ℬasic Plan

Snack Choices
Free Snack Choices

Green leafy salad with oil free vinaigrette
FUZE™ Tropical Punch Slenderize Drink-Sugar Free
Sugar Free Crystal light Beverages
Propel flavored water
Sugar Free Syfo Fruit flavored seltzers
Fresh Radishes
Herbal tea
Brewed decaf and regular coffee

Snacks under 50 calories to 75 calories

1 orange, apple or pear slices
10 fresh Lychee
1 kiwi, carambola, grapefruit, prickly pear
½ c. fresh pineapple,
1 c. papaya, strawberries or watermelon
1 guava
1 baked quince
1 c. raw celery, jicama and red pepper with low fat dip
Bristol Meyers Squib Choice Berry Almond Crisp Bar
Guilt Free Fudge Bar fat-free, sugar-free
Dole® Papaya in Peach Gel
1 c. Tropicana® Light and Healthy Orange Juice

Snacks under 100 calories

11 almonds
7 walnuts
1 lowfat string cheese
½ c. frozen jackfruit
1 frozen small banana
2 oz. Caribbean Tofu
Fat free cottage cheese with blueberries
Yoplait fat-free Strawberry Banana yogurt
Bristol Meyers Squib Diabetic Choice Vanilla or Strawberry Drink
10 Gold Mine organic mungbean chips
EAS™ AdvantEdge® low carb drink
Primal Spirit® Foods Primal Soy Strips
Del Monte Mandarin oranges-drained
¼ c. Woodstock Farms tropical fruit mix
17 Carbo LITE gummy bears

Snacks under 150 calories

1 mango, black sapote, sapodilla or pomegranate
⅓ c. Tropical hi energy trail mix
Diabetic Care Choice, Chocolate Fudge Drink
1 oz. soy nuts
¼ c. Woodstock Farms Cascade Trail Mix

Snacks under 200 calories

PowerBar® ProteinPlus™ sugar-free apple caramel bar
1 c. Stonyfield fat-free vanilla yogurt
GeniSoy® Extreme Crunch Island blast bar
Myoplex Carb Sense French Vanilla Drink

---

* 3 grams sugar-free fiber supplement

Avocado and Tomato Salsa

SERVES: 8

The strawberries really give this salsa an unusual kick! I love to serve this healthy potassium, folic acid, and vitamin-rich recipe for family or company with crunchy, cold jicama sticks.

Ingredients:

2 Florida avocados, peeled and chopped

2 fresh tomatoes, peeled, seeded, and chopped

2 tomatillo, chopped

¼ small red onion, finely chopped

1 tsp. minced garlic

½ Scotch Bonnet, seeded and chopped (use gloves when preparing to avoid capsaicin burn)

1 tbsp. key lime juice

Salt

Freshly ground black pepper

⅓ cup finely chopped cilantro

¼ cup fresh strawberries, chopped

Method:

1. Mash ½ of avocados.
2. Combine first six ingredients (except the fresh herbs). Mix until well blended. Do not crush the avocado
3. Add herbs just before serving. Taste and adjust seasonings as desired.
4. Delicately blend in fresh strawberries.
5. Serve with baked tortilla chips or raw veggies such as carrots, cucumbers, jicama and red pepper.

Chef Michelle's Tips

Like most fruits at the grocery store, avocados are primarily found unripe. To speed up the ripening process, like plantains, place in paper bag. When selecting an avocado, pick one that is blemish free and heavy for size.

Nutrition Nugget

Serve with fresh jicama, carrot, or cucumber sticks.
Also delicious with baked tortilla chips

Tropical Diet Food Servings: ½ cup veggies, 1½ fats

Baked Quince

SERVES: 1

This recipe reminds me of the traditional baked apple; however, the quince remains firmer in the serving dish than the apple. Dress up this low-cal, vitamin C, and potassium-fortified dessert with a tablespoon of dried, diced papaya to add a little color.

The rose water adds a delightful fresh, floral flavor. It's worth the hike to a specialty store to purchase a bottle or two, which you can use for rice, baked goods, and for other dishes.

Quince was considered a symbol of love by the Romans and was given to the lover as a sign of commitment, so get ready for a serious and romantic evening!

Ingredients:

1 quince
Pam spray
⅛ c. rosewater
½ tsp. cinnamon
2 tbsp. currants

Garnish (optional)
Fresh mint leaf or edible flower

Nutrition Nugget

Use ½ quince and ½ pears instead of apples in an apple pie recipe and ½ tsp. ginger, ¼ tsp. ground cloves and 1 tsp. lemon peel instead of apple pie spices.

Method:

1. Preheat oven to 375° F.
2. Quarter the quince. Core and remove seeds.
3. Place the quince in a baking tin which has been sprayed with Pam.
4. Spray just enough Pam on quince to create a shine.
5. Pour rose water over quince.
6. Sprinkle with cinnamon.
7. Cover with tinfoil and bake for 20 minutes.
8. Sprinkle with currants and cover tin with tinfoil until ready to eat.
9. Garnish with fresh mint leaf or edible flower.
10. Serve on a large Swiss chard leaf or on a colorful serving plate.

Chef Michelle's Tips

The quince season is October to December.
Look for a large yellow, firm fruit with little or no green.

Tropical Diet Food Servings: 1½ fruits

Fruit Muffin Collage
SERVES: 12

Banana, apple, and orange ingredients boost the vitamin C, fiber, and potassium content of these muffins and the fiber to give you a nutritional, morning blast or afternoon kick!

Ingredients:

2½ c. all-purpose flour
1½ c. quick cooking rolled oats
1 c. wheat germ
¾ c. granulated white sugar
2 tbsp. baking powder
½ tsp. salt
1 c. raisins

1 med. unpeeled baking apple, chopped
½ c. Egg Beaters™
1 c. ripe bananas, mashed
1 c. nonfat vanilla yogurt
2 tbsp. grated orange rind
½ c. fortified orange juice
⅓ c. Smuckers baking fat substitute

Method:

1. Preheat oven to 400°F.
2. In a large bowl, combine flour, oats, wheat germ, sugar, baking powder, and salt.
3. Stir in raisins, and apple.
4. In another bowl, whisk egg substitute lightly.
5. Blend in bananas, yogurt, orange rind, and juice and Smuckers.
6. Pour liquids into dry ingredients, stirring just until moistened.
7. Spoon about 1/3 cup batter into 12 greased or paper-lined muffin cups.
8. Bake for about 20 minutes or until firm to the touch.
9. Cool in pan for five minutes.
10. Remove from tins and cool on rack.
11. Store in airtight container if freezing.

Tropical Diet Food Servings: 1½ starches, 1 fruit

Black Beans with Tomato and Bell Pepper

SERVES: 16, ½ CUP SERVINGS

Comfort Latin-style staple food with a phytochemical kick from the tomatoes and pepper. Delicious served with warm rice, warm tostadas, and a mixed vegetable salad or with baked tortilla chips. Low carbohydrates tortilla is also available to cut the carb content of this meal.

Ingredients:

12 c. water
5 c. dried or canned organic
   black beans
1 small red onion, chopped
1 red bell pepper, chopped
1 tbsp. ground cumin
3 large bay leaves

4 c. chopped tomatoes
1 small onion, chopped
½ c. chopped garlic
1 fresh cilantro bunch, chopped
Pam Spray

Method:

1. Boil 6 c. water.
2. Add beans and cook at medium heat for 30 minutes.
3. Drain in colander and remove foreign particles.
4. Return beans to pot.
5. Add 6 c. water to beans.
6. Add red onion, bell pepper, cumin, and bay leaves and bring to boil.
7. Reduce heat to medium and cook until beans are tender, stirring occasionally.
8. Sauté tomatoes, onion, garlic and season in Pam sprayed large frying pan.
9. Drain and add beans to mixture. Turn off heat and remove from stove.
10. Transfer to bowl, serving plate or dish. Season with fresh cilantro.

Chef Michelle's Tips

If you use canned beans, you can skip the method steps 1 to 7. Just sauté the vegetables, and add cilantro. And, if you're not worried about fat and calories, in traditional Caribbean style, you add a splash of virgin olive oil at the end of the cooking process.

Tropical Diet Food Servings: 2 starches, 1 c. veggies

Boiled Plantains
SERVES: 2 TO 4

A great side dish for Grilled Swordfish recipe on page 193. A good substitution for any dish that calls for a side dish of starch.

Ingredients:

1 Semi-ripe plantain   Salt to taste
Boiling water

Methods:
1. Cut plantain into quarters.
2. Boil in skin for approximately 6 minutes.
3. Remove from water. Cool slightly.
4. Peel skin.
5. While it doesn't need any seasoning, since lightly sweet taste complements spicy main courses, you can add a bit of salt.

Tropical Diet Food Servings: 1 to 2 starches

Brocco Consommé with Leek and Garlic with a roasted pine nut hat

SERVES: 4

An easy-to-prepare, phytochemical-rich, cholesterol lowering treat! Serve in large, Mexican-style Margarita glasses for a great presentation. Inspired by Chef Goble, Sandals Resorts.

Ingredients:
4 c. organic or canned low-sodium vegetable stock 8 oz.
Broccoflower, hand-broken into small florets
1 fingernail worth of unsalted butter
2 tbsp. pine nuts, roasted
1 c. leek, chopped
4 garlic cloves, finely chopped
Salt and pepper to taste

Method:
1. Bring stock to boil. Set aside.
2. Sauté broccoflower, butter and pine nuts and add the stock.
3. Sweat leek and garlic in steamer on very low heat.
4. Add stock to sauté pan.
5. Season with black pepper. Add salt only if stock unsalted.

Chef Michelle's Tips
Broccoflower is a cross between a broccoli and cauliflower. It looks like a pale green cauliflower. Cauliflower can be substituted for this ingredient.

Tropical Diet Food Servings: 1 c. veggies, 1 fat

Miami-Style Black Bean Soup

SERVES: FOUR, 1-CUP SERVINGS

A Miami staple lunch, snack or dinner menu item. One of the first foods gringos, a slang word used to describe non-Latins, are willing to try on their first venture to a cafetería, a Latin version of the American cafeteria.

Ingredients:

Pam spray
2 oz. onion, chopped
2 garlic cloves
1 pinch coriander
2 oz. chili powder*
1 pinch cumin
2 pints chicken stock, skimmed, equal
    to 4 cups
4 oz. black beans, canned, organic best
2 tsp. soft brown sugar
4 fl. oz. red wine vinegar

Alternative Ingredients

Fat-free sour cream
2 tsp. chopped scallions

*You can use Scotch Bonnet peppers
    for a smokey chili flavor
    (see method page 193)

Method:

1. Sauté onions and garlic in pan sprayed with Pam spray.
2. Add coriander, chili power, and cumin.
3. Add stock, beans, sugar, and vinegar.
4. Garnish with a dollop of fat-free sour cream and chopped scallions. (Alternative)

✎ *Chef Michelle's Tips* ────

Use smoky chili flavor method on page 193. Serve with cut, baked, fat-free tortillas, Alvarado Street™ organic whole-wheat tortillas, or corn tortillas. Just preheat your oven to 350° F. Place tortilla flat on rack for about 5 minutes until lightly toasted. Sprinkle with kosher salt. ────

Tropical Diet Food Servings: 1 starch, ½ fat

Caribbean Ginger Chicken
SERVES: 4 TO 6

A big family hit, however start the food preparation process 3 hours in advance of mealtime.

Ingredients:

juice and zest of 1 key lime or 1 tbsp. key lime juice
juice of 1 Florida orange
1 tbsp. honey
2 tbsp. grated fresh ginger
4 cloves garlic, minced
½ tsp. cinnamon
1 tsp. pepper sauce or ground fresh pepper
4 4-oz. skinless, boneless chicken breasts

Pam vegetable spray
1 8 oz. can organic or regular canned tomatoes, crushed with juices
kosher salt and fresh ground pepper to taste

Garnish (optional)
Mandarin oranges

Method

1. Combine the lime juice, orange juice, and honey. Add ginger, garlic, cinnamon, and pepper sauce.
2. Add marinade to chicken pieces and rub well. Cover and refrigerate for 2 hours.
3. Heat the Pam in a large sauté pan. Add the chicken pieces, one at a time, reserving the marinade, and brown on each side.
4. Pour on reserved marinade, add the tomatoes and lime zest.
5. Season with kosher salt and freshly ground black pepper.
6. Cover and simmer until cooked, about 20 minutes, turning pieces occasionally.
7. Remove the chicken pieces, increase the heat on the pan and reduce juices to a nicely thickened sauce. Pour over chicken and serve.
8. Garnish with mandarin orange sections.

Chef Michelle's Tips

The local Miami community uses sour orange with lime as marinade. It's grown locally, not good to eat, but gives a wonderful flavor to chicken and pork. It can be bought bottled or fresh squeezed. Use one or two for this recipe.

Tropical Diet Food Servings: 4 protein, ½ vegetable

Gingered Papaya Muffins
SERVES: 12

A delightful blend of vitamin C and A, potassium rich and colorful blend to give you a morning or afternoon kick. Inspired by the Quick & Healthy Cookbook.

Ingredients:

1 c. all-purpose flour	½ tsp. baking powder
¾ c. whole wheat flour	2 6-oz. jars baby food carrots
¾ c. white sugar	½ c. Egg Beaters™
½ c. oat bran	½ c. papaya, pureed
1 tsp. baking soda	¼ c. currants
1 tsp. allspice, cinnamon, or nutmeg	½ tsp. fresh chopped ginger
½ tsp. salt (optional)	½ tbsp. chopped ginger

Method:

1. Preheat oven to 350° degrees.
2. Spray muffin tins with Pam.
3. In a medium bowl, combine flours, sugar, oat bran, baking soda, baking powder, spices, and salt.
4. In a large bowl, mix carrots, egg substitute, papaya, currants, and ginger.
5. Stir flour mixture into papaya mixture just until moistened.
6. Spoon batter into muffin tins.
7. Bake for 26 minutes or until toothpick inserted in the center comes out clean.

Tropical Diet Food Servings: 2 starch, ½ fruit

Ceviche Key Lime Shot

SERVES: 4

A fun appetizer to prepare and present by Chef Michelle.

Ingredients:

2 fresh key limes
2 oz. scallop, very fresh
2 oz. conch, very fresh
4 tsp. fresh ginger, grated

2 oz. spring onion—finely chopped
⅛ tsp. Scotch Bonnet peppers, grated
⅛ tsp. coriander

Method:

1. Scoop the flesh from two fresh key limes. Reserve shells and place juice aside in bowl with all Ceviche ingredients.
2. Place in refrigerator 6 hours or overnight to marinate. The lime juice actually cooks the protein in the scallop and conch.
3. Fill each key lime half with ceviche.
4. Great for company, guests can "shoot" the ceviche by squeezing the key lime.

Chef Michelle's Tips

Use very fresh seafood, conch can be very tough when not fresh. Pompano, red snapper, or sole also good substitutes, or imitation shrimp for vegetarians.

Tropical Diet Food Servings: 1 protein

Chef Michelle's Island-Style Chicken Wrap

SERVES 4

Great appetizer

Ingredients:

4 oz. skinless and boneless chicken
   breast
1 tsp. jerk seasoning
1 key lime
4 oz. arugula
1 red pepper—cut into strips
4 nonfat flour tortilla halves
1 oz. salsa

Optional:
For low-carb diets, use low-carb
   tortilla, steamed lettuce, or
   Swiss chard leaf.

Method:

1. Brush chicken breast with jerk seasoning and squeeze key lime over top.
2. Grill in medium to hot large frying pan sprayed with Pam.
3. Slice grilled chicken breast and divide into 1 oz. servings.
4. Take tortilla half and place 1 oz. chicken, 1 oz. arugula, a few red pepper strips, and roll into tortilla.
5. Seal with decorative toothpick in center.
6. Serve with a dab of salsa.
7. You can multiply this recipe for family or company.

Tropical Diet Food Servings: 1 protein, ¼ starch

Cinnamon Tuna Steak

SERVES: 4

A unique combination of flavors, perfectly complimented with a side of steamed broccoli, carrot, and cauliflower bouquet. A protein and omega-3 dietary boost! Inspired by Chef Lee Goble, Sandals Resorts.

Ingredients:

Pam vegetable cooking spray
4 3-oz. tuna steaks
1 tsp. cinnamon
1 tsp. coriander
¼ oz. key lime juice

½ lime rind

Garnish (optional)
Fresh parsley

Method:

1. Rub tuna with cinnamon and coriander.
2. Squeeze lime juice over steak.
3. In a very hot, Pam sprayed, large skillet, fry steaks.
4. Sear each side and cook as long as you like, seconds for rare, or longer.

Chef Michelle's Tips

So many tunas, so little time . . . which one is which? Tuna is seasonal from late spring to early fall. Sushi tuna is a yellow fin tuna (ahi), known for its pink color. Bluefin tuna is dark red. Albacore is what you find in canned tuna. You can buy tuna fresh or frozen, in steak, or filet form. This dish calls for a steak. Always buy your tuna fresh, and choose center-cut pieces.

Tropical Diet Food Servings: 1½ protein, ½ fat

Chef Michelle's Crème Fraiche
SERVINGS: AS NEEDED

You can take a short-cut, and buy it at a gourmet market.

Ingredients:
1 c. whipping cream
2 tbsp. buttermilk

Alternative:
Lite or non-fat whipping creme

Method:
1. Combine cream and buttermilk in glass container.
2. Cover and set at room temperature (air conditioned) for 8 to 24 hours. It will become very thick.
3. Can be refrigerated up to 10 days.

Tropical Diet Food Servings: Too many fat servings! 2 tbsp. = 2 fat

Christophene Gratin

SERVE: 6 TO 8

Christophene is the island term for the chayote vegetable. It's also known as cho-cho. This dish is the perfect complement to any fish or chicken dish. The tomatoes and fresh parsley kick-up the color.

Ingredients:

1 lb. ripe tomatoes, firm
3 lb. chayote
½ tsp. salt
Pam vegetable cooking spray
½ c. dry Italian breadcrumbs
½ c. fresh parsley chopped
1 tsp. fresh oregano

1 tsp. freshly ground black pepper
½ c. chicken broth, organic, or low-sodium, canned
2 tbsp. low-fat Parmesan cheese
1 tsp. garlic, minced

Method:

1. Preheat oven to 350° F.
2. Slice tomatoes into ¼ inch thick slices.
3. Peel chayote. Slice in half lengthways, and then slice into ¼ inch thick slices. Steam with a little salt for 5 minutes. Drain.
4. Mix together the breadcrumbs, parsley, oregano, pepper, Parmesan, and garlic. Spray lightly with Pam.
5. Lightly grease a casserole dish with Pam spray.
6. Place a row of christophene, then a row of breadcrumbs then a row of tomatoes in the dish.
7. Continue overlapping the veggies and breadcrumbs until all of them are used.
8. Drizzle broth over vegetable layers.
9. Sprinkle with Parmesan cheese.
10. Bake for 30-minutes until top is browned, but vegetables are still firm.
11. You can also bake it at higher temperature and use thinner slices for tighter casserole.

Tropical Diet Food Servings: 1 cup veggies, ¼ starch, ½ fat

Citrus Chicken

SERVES: 6

This chicken is delicious as a main course, in salads, or as sandwich filler. The fresh rosemary is on the aphrodisiac list so don't be surprised if, well. . . . Adapted from the Krome Avenue Cookbook.

Ingredients:

½ c. Tropicana® Light èn orange juice
1½ tbsp. key lime juice
1 tbsp. extra virgin olive oil
1 tbsp. fresh rosemary leaves or
    1 teaspoon dried

¼ tsp. freshly ground black pepper
3 4-oz. skinless, boneless chicken
    breasts
kosher salt to taste

Method:

1. Combine the orange and lime juices, olive oil, rosemary, and pepper. Beat together until blended.
2. Cut the chicken breasts in halves and place in a heavy self-sealing bag.
3. Add the marinade, mix well, seal the bag, and refrigerate at least 2 hours, and up to 10 hours.
4. Drain the chicken. Place on a moderately hot grill. Or in oven broiler. Grill until browned, turning only to cook evenly. About 20 minutes.
5. When done, the chicken should be golden on both sides. The juices should run clear when the meat is slit with a knife. (If thinly sliced chicken is used, check doneness after 10 minutes.)
6. Sprinkle with salt. Serve hot or at room temperature.

Chef Michelle's Tips

You can substitute rosemary, with cilantro basil. Delicious with steamed asparagus with slivered almonds.

Tropical Diet Food Servings: 2 protein, ½ fat

Confetti Corn Bread

SERVES: 12

Colorful cornbread with a phytochemical kick and a chili bite! You can use a store bought packaged corn bread, and skip the first six to eight ingredients. Don't leave out the peppers for your vitamin C boost.

Ingredients:

¼ c. red and green sweet peppers
  chopped
1¼ c. all-purpose flour
1 tbsp. baking powder
1 tbsp. sugar
½ tsp. salt
¾ c. cornmeal

¼ c. Egg Beaters™
¾ c. nonfat milk
3 tbsp. Smuckers fat substitute

Optional:
¼ Scotch or Serrano chili pepper

Method:
1. Preheat oven to 425° F.
2. Chop red and green sweet peppers.
3. Sift flour, baking powder, sugar, and salt.
4. Add cornmeal.
5. In separate bowl beat egg substitute, milk, and oil substitute together.
6. Pour liquid into dry ingredients.
7. Combine with a few gentle strokes. DO NOT OVERMIX.
8. Spoon the batter in a decorative 9" square pan.
9. Place in center of oven rack and bake for 25 minutes with a watchful eye. DO NOT BURN!

Tropical Diet Food Servings: 1½ starch, ¼ veggie

Crab, Ginger, and Grapefruit Salad
SERVES: 4

A cold and easy salad to prepare, serve on a bed of dark greens for extra folic acid. Find a decorative seashell or plate for a great presentation. Inspired by Chef Lee Goble, Sandals Resorts.

Ingredients:

8 oz. ready-to-eat crabmeat, or crabmeat vegetarian substitute, chopped
4 tsp. Dijon mustard
1 tsp. olive oil
8 tbsp. grated ginger
4 oz. lemon, grated
4 oz. lettuce, shredded
4 large green leaves
8 oz. grapefruit, fresh sections, or canned unsweetened, sliced in thirds

Method:

1. Mix crabmeat.
2. Marinate crabmeat with lemon.
3. Season with mustard, oil, and ginger.
4. Toss with shredded lettuce and grapefruit sections.
5. Serve on large green leaf on a clean seashell, decorative green doily, or plate.

Tropical Diet Food Servings: 1 protein, ½ fruit

Gingered Carrot and Pear Bisque
SERVES: 4 TO 6

A fun, fresh, and colorful soup, loaded with phytonutrients, vitamins, and minerals. Refreshing as an appetizer, main lunch course, or afternoon snack. Prepare ahead of time. Delicious hot or cold. Chef Pat Vandenberg helped this recipe come alive!

Ingredients:

1 c. diced onion
Pam vegetable cooking spray
2 pears, large unpeeled, diced
   miniscule
1 tbsp. ginger, fresh, peeled and
   minced
2 c. chicken broth, organic or
   unsalted canned
1 lb. carrots, peeled and cut
   into chunks

½ c. cooked white rice
1 bay leaf
1½ c. fat-free half & half
Salt and pepper to taste

Garnish:
Carrot shaving
Fresh dill

Method:

1. Sauté the onion in a large saucepan sprayed with Pam until the onion is translucent and tender.
2. Add ginger, and sauté another minute or two.
3. Add the chicken broth, carrots, pears, rice, and bay leaf, and simmer, partly covered, until the carrots are tender.
4. Remove the bay leaf. Puree the mixture in a blender, or food processor, blending in the fat-free cream, or half & half to thin the soup to your taste.
5. Season with salt and pepper.
6. Reheat the soup gently, and serve it hot, or let it cool completely, and place in refrigerator for 2 hours.
7. Serve cold with a garnish of carrot shaving and fresh dill.

Tropical Diet Food Servings: 1 fruit, ¼ c. starch

Island Vegetable Soup

SERVES: 6 TO 8

An easy-to-prepare, nutrient-rich comfort-stew, served warm or cool with a fresh green salad, as a meal, or as main course on its own. Can also be kept in the refrigerator for a day or two, without losing flavor.

Ingredients:

1 lb. cassava and yams, peeled, and cut into large chunks
Pam spray
1 small onion, chopped
1 red bell pepper, cut into strips
1 small chayote, peeled and diced
1 can organic or low-sodium commercial-brand chicken broth
½ c. chopped chives

2 garlic cloves, minced
2 tbsp. fresh ginger chopped
1 can (14 oz.) tomatoes with juice
1 tbsp. chopped basil
1 tbsp. fresh thyme
salt and ground pepper
1 plantain, completely ripe
3 tomatillo, chopped

Method:

1. Steam cassava and yam over high heat until tender. Remove and set aside.
2. Heat Pam in a large sauté pan, add onion, and pepper. Sauté until fragrant, about 3 minutes.
3. Add chayote and broth and cook.
4. Cover until tender, about 5 minutes.
5. Add chives, garlic, ginger and tomatoes, breaking the tomatoes with the back of spoon.
6. Then add the basil and thyme and cook covered for an additional 10 minutes over a low heat.
7. Season with salt and freshly ground black pepper.
8. Stir in steamed plantain and tomatillo.
9. Cook for about 1 to 2 minutes more.
10. Serve in clear bowls.

Chef Michelle's Tips

Plantains should be completely ripe for soup or they will get mushy and dissolve.

Tropical Diet Food Servings: 1½ starch, 1 c. veggies

Garbanzo Cake

SERVES: 10

Don't let the garbanzo beans, also known as chickpeas, scare you. It's a delicious way to get extra B-vitamins and fiber. Your loved ones will never know this cake is made from beans. Don't kiss and tell Either! The dessert is great with any meal. According to Chef Michelle, the cake would also taste good with a variety of meats, or even the Cinnamon Tuna recipe on page 181.

Ingredients:

2 10 oz. cans garbanzo beans, organic, or commercial-brand rinsed and drained
1 c. Egg Beaters™

1 c. unsweetened applesauce
1 tsp. baking powder
2 tsp. ground cinnamon
1 orange, zest with juice

Method:

1. Preheat the oven to 350° F.
2. Tip the chickpeas in a colander, drain them thoroughly, then rub them between palms of your hand to loosen and remove the skins.
3. Put the skinned chickpeas in a food processor and process until smooth.
4. Spoon the puree into a bowl and stir in the egg substitute, applesauce, baking powder, cinnamon, orange rind and juice. Use Baker's Spray to spray a loaf pan.
5. Pour the cake mixture into the pan, level the surface and bake for about 1½ hours, or until a skewer inserted into the center comes out clean.
6. Remove the cake from the oven, and let stand in the pan, for about 10 minutes.
7. Remove cake from the pan. Place on a wire rack.
8. Let cool completely before serving.
9. Serve with sliced fresh pineapple, or nonfat vanilla frozen yogurt.

Tropical Diet Food Servings: 1 starch, 1 fruit

Rose Flan

SERVES: 6

A low-fat, rosy version of this traditional Latin dessert. You'll need to prepare this at least 4 hours ahead of serving time. A personal favorite.

Ingredients:

½ c. organic sugar
¼ c. rose water
½ c. egg substitutes
3 large egg whites

1 can (14-oz.) fat-free, sweetened, condensed milk
1½ c. skim milk
1 tbsp.vanilla extract

Method:

1. Preheat oven to 325° degrees.
2. Combine sugar and rose water in a small saucepan.
3. Bring to a simmer over low heat, stirring occasionally. Increase heat to medium-high and cook, without stirring, until syrup turns a deep amber color, 5 to 8 minutes.
4. Pour syrup into a 1½ to 2 quart soufflé dish. Tilt dish to coat with syrup.
5. Whisk egg substitute and egg whites in a large bowl.
6. Blend in sweetened, fat-free condensed milk, skim milk, and vanilla. Pour egg mixture through a strainer into syrup-coated dish.
6. Bake in a water bath (another larger pan with water in it) 60 to 70 minutes. Cool to room temperature.
7. Refrigerate at least 4 hours or overnight.

Chef Michelle's Tips

Can also be served with rosemary or thyme for a savory option, as a great side to lamb or fish. Dessert substitutions include jasmine, coconut, or ginger.

Tropical Diet Food Servings:1 milk, 1 fruit

Ginger Papaya Cocktail
SERVES: 2

Morning or night, this refreshing vitamin-spiked cocktail will liven your senses and maybe even your love life ❤

Ingredients:

1 large ripe papaya, deseeded and
   peeled
Juice of 2 key limes
3 tbsp. ginger, grated

Evening Cocktail
Add 2 oz. of *Imperia*™ Vodka
   (see description on page 192)

Garnish Option
Mint leaf for garnish

Method:

1. Place papaya in food processor or blender, and puree.
2. Add lime juice and grated ginger.
3. Continue to blend.
4. Garnish with mint leaf.
5. For evening cocktail, add *Imperia*™ vodka.

Chef Michelle's Tips

This drink would also taste great infused with champagne. Papaya can be substituted with passion fruit.

Tropical Diet Food Servings: 1 fruit
With Vodka: 1 fruit, ½ fat (alcohol)

The Imperia™ Vodka Story

"There are no harmful elements, only harmful quantities."

Dimiti Mendeleev (1894)
Inventor of the Periodic Table and
creator of the Imperial standard of Russian Vodka

If you're going to drink alcohol, you might want to consider a nice tropical vodka martini. Why? The process that makes *Imperia*™ vodka velvety and pure is also scientifically *sexy*. Here's how the story goes.

Prior to the Russian Empire of Nicholas II in St. Petersburg, Russian vodka was a rough, harsh spirit. Nicholas II had a brilliant scientist at his employ—Dimitri Mendeleev, famous for inventing the Periodic Table of Elements (remember high school chemistry?). Nicholas II ordered Mendeleev to formulate a standard of vodka, that would not only eliminate the unpleasant side effects of poorly prepared vodka, but also create the Russian Standard of vodka. Mendeleev obliged.

Today, the Russian Standard company, makers of Russia's best selling premium vodkas, continue to use Mendeleev's historic formula.

You see, expertly made vodka can be one of the purest distilled spirits within the world, because vodka comes from distillates that are collected at higher temperatures, and finely filtered to eliminate most of the congeners, chemicals that cause hangovers, headaches, and dehydration. These congeners are esters, fusel oils, aldehydes, and methanol. Spirits that distill at lower temperatures, and do not use micro-filtration, leave these congeners in the resultant spirit. The worst offenders tend to be darker colored spirits.

Imperia™ vodka begins with the elegance of Mendeleev's original formula, the finest wheat grain and softest northern waters, and perfects the formula with the most modern of distillation and purification processes. The result is vodka of velvety and unmatched smoothness, and shimmering clarity.

So, relax. Enjoy a "nutritious" vitamin C–rich *Imperia*™ screwdriver—prepared with freshly squeezed or fortified orange juice, a strawberry, or pineapple-vodka martini.

Thank you to Jose Aragon for sharing the Imperia™ *vodka story.*

Grilled Swordfish With Serrano and lime sauce

SERVES: 4

Adapted from Krome Avenue Cookbook *from the Fruit and Spice Park, Homestead, Florida.*

Ingredients:

2 Serrano chilies, fresh
4 medium fresh tomatoes, firm
Pam regular cooking spray
1 key lime, zest and juice
Pam olive oil vegetable cooking spray
4 4-oz. swordfish steaks

¾ c. crème fraiche (recipe on page 182)
½ tsp. salt
½ tsp. fresh black pepper

Garnish (optional)
Fresh flat-leaf parsley or cilantro

Method:

1. Roast chilies in a dry griddle until the skins are blistered. Place in plastic baggie. Set aside.
2. Cut a cross at the bottom of each tomato. Place them in a heatproof bowl and pour in boiling water to cover. After 3 minutes, lift the tomatoes out with a slotted spoon. Plunge them into a bowl of cold water. Drain.
3. Pull the skin off, cut the tomatoes in half and squeeze out the seeds. Chop the tomato flesh into ½ inch pieces.
4. Heat the Pam regular spray in a small saucepan. Add chile strips, lime zest and juice. Cook for 2 to 3 minutes. Stir in the tomatoes. Spray with Pam as needed.
5. Cook for 10 minutes, stirring the mixture occasionally, until the tomato is pulpy.
6. Spray the swordfish steaks with Pam olive oil spray and season. Grill or pan fry for 3 to 4 minutes, or until just cooked, turning once.
7. Stir the crème fraiche into the sauce, and heat it gently.
8. Pour crème onto the swordfish steaks. Serve with fresh parsley or cilantro.

Chef Michelle's Tips

To give chilies a smoky flavor, place chilies on oven range burner. Turn on all sides until skin is blackened. Place chilies in brown paper bag until they are cool. Crème Fraiche recipe on page 182. Great side item is boiled plantains. See recipe on page 174. Another great side dish is grilled asparagus.

Tropical Diet Food Servings: 3 protein, 1 fat

Island Pork

SERVES: 2

A delicious, healthy pork dish designed for a woman's sailing camp hosted by the Bitter End Resorts in the British Virgin Islands. Designed by Chef Trevor Nicely.

Ingredients:

2 4-oz. pork tenderloins
1 tsp. fresh thyme
4 tbsp. garlic cloves, chopped
½ tsp. ground cumin
½ tsp. white pepper
2 tbsp. basil, fresh leaves
kosher salt to taste

Fruit Salsa:
2 oz. mango pieces, chopped
½ tsp. tabasco sauce
2 oz. pineapple, fresh or canned
    chopped
2 oz. red bell peppers chopped
½ tsp. cilantro fresh
2 oz. red onion, chopped

Method

1. Preheat oven to 350° F.
2. Cut slits in pork. Stuff garlic cloves inside. Flavor of roasted garlic will run through the meat. Season and set aside.
3. In the meantime, mix salsa ingredients, and place in refrigerator to set.
4. Roast the pork for 10 to15 minutes until pink of meat is gone.
5. Remove and serve with fruit salsa.

Chef Michelle's Tips

Would taste delicious with roasted corn and rice. ————————

Tropical Diet Food Servings: 3 protein, 1 fat
With Fruit Salsa: 3 protein, 1 fat, 1 fruit

Jicama Salsa

SERVES: 4

Jicama is a great, safe, low-cal tropical vegetable to try, especially if you're leery of trying some of the other unusual tropical vegetables and fruits mentioned in this book. Crunchy and delicious, this salsa will fire-up any baked tortilla chip, or fish dish.

Ingredients:

1 small red onion, chopped
Juice of 2 key limes
3 small mandarin oranges, from can,
    with about 2 tbsp. juice
1 1-lb.-jicama, diced small
½ cucumber, diced small

Optional:
1 Congo chili

Method:

1. Cut the onion in half. Dice fine.
2. Place in a bowl with key lime juice. Let soak.
3. Slice mandarin oranges.
4. Peel the jicama and rinse in cold water.
5. Cut into quarters, and then slice finely. Add to a bowl of mandarin orange juice.
6. Cut the cucumber in half longwise, and then use a teaspoon to scoop out the seeds. Slice the cucumber and add to the bowl.
7. With gloves, remove the stem from the chile, slit it and scrape out the seeds with a small sharp knife. Chop the flesh fincly and add to the bowl.
8. Add the sliced onion to the bowl, with any remaining lime juice, and mix well. Cover and let stand at room temperature for at least 1 hour before serving. If not serving, refrigerate salsa. It will keep for 2 to 3 days.

Tropical Diet Food Servings: ½ c veggies, ¼ fruit

Lychees with Strawberry Dressing
SERVE: 4

A unique use for this tropical fruit, delicious as is, or can be used as a topping or side, with other desserts.

Ingredients:

16 lychees, fresh or canned in juice
    or rinsed from syrup
5 oz. fresh strawberries or
    unsweetened frozen strawberries
1 tbsp. honey

Optional Garnish:
Fresh mint leaves

Method:

1. Place lychees in serving bowl.
2. Puree the strawberries in a blender.
3. Add honey. Blend again for about 30 seconds.
4. Dress the lychees with the strawberry puree.
5. Refrigerate until ready to serve.
6. Place in a clear martini or champagne glass.
7. Garnish with mint leaves.

Chef Michelle's Tips

Would be delicious over angel food cake. Lychees are also tasty with chocolate.

Tropical Diet Food Servings: 1 fruit

Mango Relish

SERVES: 8

According to Chris Rollins, Director for the Fruit and Spice Park, mangos are one of the healthiest fruits. This recipe is adapted from The Krome Avenue Cookbook, *available from The Fruit and Spice Park. This dish can also be cooked and used as chutney. Both are great as a side to fish, pork, or chicken dishes.*

Ingredients:

4 green mangos, large, peeled, and grated

1 onion, small, minced

1 tsp. peanut oil

1 fresh red chili pepper, seeded, deveined and diced

1 green chili pepper, seeded, deveined and diced

Salt and freshly ground black pepper to taste

Method:

1. Combine the mangos, onion, oil, and chili peppers.
2. Salt and pepper to taste.
3. Cover and refrigerate for at least 2 hours.
4. Serve the relish fresh. It will keep for 2 to 3 days in the refrigerator

Tropical Diet Food Servings: ½ fruit

Papaya Morning Muffins

SERVES: 8 TO 12

Nutritious, easy to make, and delicious to eat any time of day.

Ingredients:

1 box Canterbury Cuisine pumpkin
   cake mix

½ c. Egg Beaters™
1¼ c. fresh papaya, chopped

Method:

1. Preheat oven to 375° F.
2. In a large bowl, combine all ingredients, and stir until blended (liquid not needed in preparation).
3. Spoon into greased or paper lined muffin pan.
4. Bake for approximately 23 minutes.
5. Let cool for 5 minutes.

Chef Michelle's Tips

A lot of people in the Miami community take papaya juice in the morning to aid with digestion. Papaya puree also makes a good vinaigrette.

Tropical Diet Food Servings: 1 starch, ½ fruit

Tropical Hot Mango Salsa

SERVES: 6 ½-CUP SERVINGS

Feeling hot,hot,hot. Tangy, tingling salsa. Excellent with snapper.

Ingredients:

2 mangos, half-ripe, finely chopped
1 garlic clove, minced
1 Congo pepper, seeded and finely
  chopped, more-or-less to taste
1 tbsp. key lime juice, fresh or bottled
4 tbsp. cilantro, fresh, finely chopped

3 red peppers, mini, or ¼ large red
  peppers, chopped
Salt and freshly ground black pepper
  to taste

Method:

1. Combine mangos, garlic, Congo pepper, and red pepper, and key lime juice.
2. Add salt and pepper to taste.
3. Let stand for 1-hour before serving.
4. Add the fresh cilantro just before serving.

Tropical Diet Food Servings: 1 fruit

Mango, Strawberry and Christophene Salad
SERVES: 8

A delightful blend of tropical fruits and chayote vegetable—great accompaniment to any meal, or side dish to fish, chicken or meat.

Ingredients:

2 c. fresh strawberries, sliced
1 chayote, medium, cut into ¼-inch cubes
1 mango, large, peeled and cut into ¼-inch cubes
8 c. mixed torn salad greens

Dressing:
⅓ c. rice wine vinegar
1 tbsp. walnut oil
1 tbsp. granulated white sugar
1½ tbsp. fresh mint, chopped
¼ tsp. salt and pepper to taste

Method:

1. In a large bowl, whisk together vinegar, oil, sugar, mint, salt and pepper.
2. Add strawberries, christophene and mango.
3. Top greens with strawberry, mango and christophene mixture.
4. Divide greens among 8 clear plates.

Tropical Diet Food Servings: 1 fruit, 1 fat

Mango Madness Cocktail

SERVES: 2

A delicious way to nutricize your evening cocktail with vitamins A, C, and potassium.

Ingredients:

2 ripe mangos
4 oz. vanilla low-fat yogurt
4 oz. Tropicana® Orange Juice
Ice
2 oz. *Imperia*™ vodka to taste

Low-calorie substitutions:
Tropicana® Light orange juice
Non-fat vanilla yogurt

Method:

1. Peel mango.
2. Place mango in food processor with yogurt, orange juice, ice and *Imperia*™ vodka.
3. Serve with an orange twist garnish

◉ *Nutrition Nugget*

To save calories and carbohydrate grams use Tropicana® Light orange juice. To save fat grams, use non-fat vanilla yogurt.

Tropical Diet Food Servings: 2 fruit, ¼ milk, 1 fat (alcohol)

Pasta Tropical

SERVES: 8

A colorful dish I created years ago. It has been featured in numerous magazines.

Ingredients:

16 oz. tricolor or sport-shaped pasta like bicycle, tennis rackets, etc.— cooked, drained and cooled, no salt used in cooking

1 c. frozen peas, no-salt added, thawed

1 c. corn, canned or frozen, no-salt added

1 c. garbanzo beans, organic or regular rinsed

¼ c. raisins

1 c. mandarin oranges, canned in juice, or lite syrup and drained

Dressing
1 tbsp. canola or lite "flavorful" oil like walnut oil
3 tbsp. fortified orange juice
1 tsp. cinnamon
¼ tsp. ginger, fresh
¼ tsp. nutmeg
¼ tsp. orange peel, grated

Method:

1. Cook pasta according to directions. Remove from heat, rinse, and drain.
2. Cool pasta in refrigerator for approximately 10 to 15 minutes. Remove.
3. Toss in peas, corn, garbanzo beans, and raisins.
4. Prepare dressing by combining oil and spices thoroughly.
5. Toss pasta and dressing.
6. Garnish with mandarin oranges.
7. Serve with fresh green salad.

Tropical Diet Food Servings: 2 starch, ½ protein, 1 fruit, ½ fat

Pineapple-Onion Salsa

SERVES: 14 ½-CUP SERVINGS

Adapted from Krome Avenue Cookbook *from The Fruit and Spice Park, a delicious salsa twist, and tasty served with baked tortilla chips.*

Ingredients:

1 pineapple, fresh, finely chopped, or 1 large can pineapple in its own juice, chopped

1 sweet onion, finely chopped

6 tbsp. fresh mint, minced

2 tbsp. serrano or jalapeno chilies, minced

salt and fresh ground pepper to taste

Option:
baked, low-fat tortilla chips.

Method

1. Mix first 4 ingredients in large bowl.
2. Season with salt and pepper.
3. Chill up to 8 hours.
4. Serve with baked store bought tortilla chips or make them fresh yourself.

Chef Michelle's Tips

Can grill or roast pineapple for different flavor—Vidalia onion would be great.

Tropical Diet Food Servings: ⅓ fruit

Pomegranate Morning Cocktail

SERVES: 2

A stimulating morning-beverage rich in vitamin C. Also creates an exotic, evening cocktail.

Ingredients for morning cocktail:

    2 pomegranates
    4 oz. flavored seltzer
    1 tbsp. sugar
    2 orange slices, fresh

Evening Cocktail Add:

    2 oz. Bacardi White Rum or
    2 oz. white wine

Method:

    1. Strain (or extract) the pomegranate juice.
    2. Pour into jug with citrus seltzer and oranges.
    3. Pour into tall highball glasses (over ice for evening.)
    4. Slit the orange, and hang over side of glass.

Chef Michelle's Tips

Pomegranates have a short season in the United States—October to November. Choose heavy and bright pomegranates. Good substitution for pomegranates is passion fruit. Fruit can be refrigerated up to 2 months. Could also add wine to original mix, and have pomegranate white wine spritzer.

Tropical Diet Food Servings
Morning Juice: 2 fruits
Evening Cocktail: 2 fruits, 1 fat (alcohol)

Roasted Green Beans and Pepper

SERVES: 4

A phytochemical-rich dish, ideal for a side to red meat, pork, seafood, or poultry dishes. Adapted from the Krome Avenue Cookbook, *Fruit and Spice Park.*

Ingredients:

¾ lb. green beans, fresh, ends trimmed, cut diagonally into halves

1 red bell pepper, large, cut into long thin strips

1 green bell, large pepper diced

Pam olive oil vegetable spray

½ tsp. Creole seasoning

1 tsp. Mrs. Dash seasoning

Method:

1. Preheat oven broiler to 450° F.
2. Place green beans and peppers on a baking sheet. Spread the vegetables in an even layer.
3. Spray veggies with Pam olive oil spray.
4. Mix seasoning and season veggies evenly.
5. Roast for about 12 minutes or until the vegetables are browned and tender.
6. Stir midway through the roasting.

Tropical Diet Food Servings: 1 c. veggies

Shrimp and Vegetable Skewer

SERVES: 4

An easy-to-prepare and present grilled or pan fry version of this island favorite.

Ingredients:

12 oz. shrimp, medium, very fresh
4 oz. red onion, diced large
1 oz. yellow pepper, diced large
1 oz. cherry tomato, whole
1 oz. tomatillo
Pam vegetable spray
Metal skewers

Dip Ingredients:

½ c. non-fat plain yogurt
2 tbsp. fresh chives
salt and fresh black pepper to taste or
seasoning of your choice, e.g., curry or
onion powder

Method:
1. Place shrimp and vegetables in an alternating pattern on skewer.
2. Spray with Pam vegetable spray.
3. Grill until shrimp is pink, and vegetables are lightly browned.
4. Prepare yogurt dip with seasoning to taste.
5. Serve on platter for the family, or for company.

Tropical Diet Food Servings: 1 1/2 protein, 1/2 c. veggies

Shrimp Sauteed with Carambola

SERVES: 4

A great way to incorporate starfruit, a vitamin C and mineral-rich fruit. Adapted from the Krome Avenue Cookbook, *Fruit and Spice Park.*

Ingredients:

3 carambola, medium-sweet
Pam vegetable cooking spray
16 oz. shrimp, small, very fresh or
    frozen

kosher salt and white pepper to taste
pinch white sugar
1 tbsp. lemon juice
½ tsp. butter

Method:

1. Cut tips off carambola. Slice fruit crosswise, ⅛-inch thick.
2. Heat Pam spray in a large sauté pan. Use anything but aluminum pan.
3. Add shrimp, carambola slices, salt, white pepper, and sugar.
4. Sauté for a couple of minutes, until shrimp are just pink.
5. Add the lemon juice and toss with the shrimp.
6. Remove from the heat and stir in ½ tsp. of butter.
7. Taste for seasoning and adjust as desired.
8. Serve at once.

Chef Michelle's Tips

Serve with avocado or tomato slices, or onion salad. These ingredients complement the sharpness of the dish.

Tropical Diet Food Servings: 2 protein, ½ fruit

Spaghetti Squash with Red Sauce
SERVES: 4

A personal favorite, easy-to-make, low-carb alternative to traditional spaghetti.

Ingredients:

1 spaghetti squash—large, heavy for weight
2 cloves fresh garlic, chopped
1 small red onion, chopped fine

PAM spray
1 jar red tomato sauce—your favorite brand, *just watch the fat content!*

Method:

1. Boil squash whole for 20 to 30 minutes. Remove and cool.
2. Remove skin, scoop out seeds, remove spaghetti guts, and separate. Spray with Pam spray to prevent sticking. Set aside.
3. Sauté onion and garlic in Pam sprayed pan, until garlic is browned, and onion is semisoft, and translucent.
4. Add bottled tomato sauce to onion and garlic. Sauté and cook at low heat for another 10 to 15 minutes or until sauce is reduced by ¼.
5. Pour over spaghetti squash, or reserve in sauce dish.
6. Sprinkle with low-fat Parmesan cheese.

◉ *Nutrition Nugget*
Can be served with lean meatballs, or Gimme Lean brand soy-protein meatballs, if you are vegetarian.

Tropical Diet Food Servings: 1½ starch,1 fat

Tropical Fruit Pancakes

SERVES: 14

A family favorite, the pancakes are loaded with tasty, naturally-sweet surprises, and lots of hidden vitamins, minerals and fibers. Serve with Warm Fruit Sauce on page 210. Adapted from the Secrets of Cooking for Long Life Cookbook, *by Sandra Woodruff, R.D.*

Ingredients:

1½ c. whole wheat pastry flour
1 tbsp. baking powder
¾ c. nonfat milk
1 c. non-fat vanilla yogurt, or plain
    non-fat yogurt with 1 tbsp. vanilla
    added
2 egg whites, lightly beaten, or ¼ c.
    fat-free egg substitute
¾ c. blueberries, fresh or frozen unsweetened

¼ c. persimmon
½ c. papaya or ½ c. kiwi
½ c. strawberries, fresh or frozen
    unsweetened
¾ c. blueberries, fresh or frozen
    unsweetened

Garnish:
Strawberry "fan"

Method:

1. Place the flour and baking powder in a large bowl. Stir to mix well.
2. Add milk, yogurt, and egg whites or egg substitute.
3. Mix with a wire whisk to blend well. Fold in the fruit combination of your choice.
4. Spray your griddle with Pam vegetable cooking spray.
5. Preheat over medium heat until a drop of water sizzles when it hits the surface.
6. For each pancake, ladle ¼ c. of the batter onto the griddle in a 2 to 4 in. circle. Cook for about 1½ minutes, or until the top is bubbly and the edges are dry. Turn and cook for an additional minute, or until the second side is golden brown.
7. As the pancakes are done, transfer to a decorative serving plate.
8. Serve hot with honey, maple syrup, warm fruit topping, lite pancake syrup, natural fruit toppings, or tropical fruit toppings and a sprinkle of powdered sugar.

Tropical Diet Food Servings: 1 starch, 1 fruit

Warm Tropical Fruit Sauce

SERVES: ABOUT 4 ¼-C. SERVINGS

Great with the Tropical Fruit Pancakes recipe on page 209, ready-to-serve waffles, or as fruit salad dip. Adapted from Secrets of Cooking for Long Life Cookbook *by registered dietitian Sandra Woodruff, R.D. (see references).*

Ingredients:

¾ c. strawberry and kiwi nectar (any tropical fruit nectar will work.)

2 c. of the following combined:
1 kiwi
¼ c. papaya
1 c. strawberries, fresh or frozen unsweetened

or

1 c. blueberries, fresh or frozen unsweetened
¼ c. strawberry, dried
¾ c. papaya
¼ c. sugar

Method:

1. Set aside 2 tbsp. of the nectar.
2. Place the remaining juice, fruit, and the sugar in a 1½ qt. saucepan. Bring to a boil over a medium to high heat. Stir to mix well.
3. Reduce heat to low, cover, and simmer for about 5 minutes, stirring occasionally.
4. Cook, for another minute or two, stirring constantly, or until the mixture is thickened and bubbly.
5. Serve warm over pancakes, French toast, or waffles.
6. Store any leftover sauce in the refrigerator for up to three days.

Tropical Diet Food Servings: 1 fruit

Tropical Mougrabiya Garden of Eden
SERVES: 8

A favorite of mine, it's an ideal vegetarian main course, and perfect with a side salad and steamed veggies. I love the size of the Mougrabiya "pellets," and the fragrance of the dish when prepared with orange blossom water. The veggies on the ingredient list add iron, calcium, vitamin C, and folic acid-rich vegetables, but any veggies will be healthy. And for the mougrabiya and orange blossom water, each can be substituted with any starch grain and broth, respectively.

Ingredients:

2 c. bottled water	1 Swiss chard leaf, chopped
⅛ c. orange blossom water*	¼ c. green peas, frozen, thawed
1 c. Lebanese Mougrabiya*	¼ c. corn, frozen niblets, thawed
3 beets, raw, peeled, diced	2 oz. anise, fresh
3 tbsp. ginger root, chopped	dash kosher salt

* Available at specially Lebanese or Middle Eastern markets. Mougrabiya imported by American Blue Mills, San Francisco, California

Method:

1. Heat water and orange blossom water until boiling in deep skillet pan.
2. Add mougrabiya, beets and ginger, mix ingredients.
3. Reduce heat and cook for 10 minutes until liquid is almost completely removed. Mix every 2 to 3 minutes.
4. Add anise, peas, and corn. Mix and cook until anise is almost clear, and the corn and peas are cooked.
5. Add a dash of kosher salt. Mix entire dish and remove from stove.
6. Serve in attractive casserole.

Tropical Diet Food Servings: 3 starch, ½ vegetable

Tropical Tres Leche
SERVES: 10 TO 12

Nutritious, high-calcium, low-fat version of this traditionally high-fat, Latin dessert. The tropical fruit adds oodles of minerals and vitamins.

Ingredients:

1 angel food cake mix
1 c. kiwi—fresh, firm, skin
   removed, chopped

Topping:
1 c. strawberries, fresh
1 c. mandarin oranges, canned in juice,
   drained

Tres Leche:
10 fl. oz. nonfat milk
10 fl. oz. nonfat condensed milk
10 fl. oz. nonfat evaporated milk

Method:

1. Preheat oven to 400° F.
2. Prepare angel food cake as per recipe on box.
3. Pour angel food cake mix into glass bowl.
4. Add 1¼ c. cool water to mix.
5. Stir until batter is completely moist.
6. Add chopped kiwi. Blend.
7. Pour into 8 x 10 glass cake pan. Bake for 30 minutes until cake is slightly brown, and a clean knife can be stuck in, and pulled out of the center of the cake.
8. Remove from oven.
9. Let cake cool for 10 minutes to ½ hour.
10. Place in refrigerator for 30 minutes. Remove.
11. Garnish and serve without tres leche or . . .
12. Stab the cake with knives in rows and columns without destroying the integrity of the cake shape.
13. Mix tres leches, the three milks in glass bowl.
14. Pour slowly over entire cake, making sure all parts of cake are covered.
15. Refrigerate for 30 minutes to 1-hour. Remove from refrigerator.
16. Decorate cake in pattern with sliced strawberries and mandarin oranges. You can also use grape halves, fresh berries or any other non-runny fruit of your choice.

Tropical Diet Food Servings: 2 starches, 2 fruits
With tres leche: 2 starches, 2 fruits, 1 milk serving

Vegetarian Chili

SERVES: 4

From my book, The Vegetarian Sports Nutrition Guide *(Wiley, 2000).*

Ingredients:

½ onion, diced
1 red pepper, diced
1 green pepper, diced
Pam olive oil vegetable spray
3 c. tomatoes, fresh, chopped small
1 c. V-8 vegetable juice
2 tbsp. cumin
2 tbsp. chili powder
1 bay leaf
¼ c. texturized vegetable protein (TVP), available at health food stores
2 c. vegetable stock, organic, or low-sodium, canned

1 15-oz. can kidney beans, organic, or commercial-brand, rinsed
Salt and pepper to taste

Optional:
2 jalapenos, fresh, diced

Garnish:
Chopped chives.
Shredded fat-free cheddar cheese

Method:

1. Sauté diced vegetables in a pan sprayed with Pam spray.
2. Add tomatoes. Stew for 5 minutes. Add V-8 juice and continue to simmer.
3. Add seasoning and bay leaf.
4. Add TVP and allow to absorb tomato coloring and flavor.
5. Add stock and beans. Toss in diced jalapenos if desired.
6. Simmer on low heat for 3 minutes.
7. Remove bay leaf.
8. Ladle into separate soup bowls or large coffee mugs.
9. Garnish with a pinch of chopped chives and fat-free cheddar cheese.

Tropical Diet Food Servings: 1½ protein, 2½ cups veggies, 1 fat

Vegetable Lasagna
SERVES: 6

A low-carb, low-calorie, spin-off of the classic dish—this layered creation was adapted from the Krome Avenue Cookbook *and perfected by Chef Pat Vandenberg.*

Ingredients:

Pam vegetable cooking spray
½ eggplant, medium, trimmed, thinly sliced lengthwise
¼ tsp. salt
¼ tsp. white pepper
1 tbsp. garlic, minced
¼ c. low-fat Parmesan cheese
2 sweet onions, medium, thinly-sliced

1 zucchini squash, medium, trimmed, thinly-sliced, lengthwise
1 yellow squash, medium, trimmed, thinly-sliced, lengthwise
¼ c. fat-free mozzarella cheese
4 tomatoes, fresh, firm, thinly-sliced
1½ tbsp. fresh parsley, minced

Method:

1. Preheat oven to 325° F. Spray the bottom and sides of a glass 8x10-in. casserole baking dish.
2. Cover the bottom of dish with slightly overlapping eggplant slices.
3. Sprinkle this layer with ¼ teaspoon each of salt and pepper, some of the garlic and Parmesan.
4. Top this with a layer of slightly overlapping onion slices and then a layer of zucchini.
5. Season again. This time add some mozzarella.
6. Continue layering the tomatoes, zucchini, and then tomatoes again.
7. Season. Press down with your hand on lasagna to compact the layers. Drain any liquid.
8. Finish with a layer of slightly overlapping tomatoes, and a layer of eggplant. Finish with the seasoning, cheese, and parsley.
9. Cover with foil, and bake for 15 minutes.
10. Remove foil and bake until lightly brown, about another 10 to 15 minutes. Remove from oven.
11. Carefully using oven gloves, tilt dish and pour off the excess liquid.
12. Serve either warm or at room temperature.

Tropical Diet Food Servings: 1 cup veggies, ½ protein or ½ dairy (cheese)

Chicken Salad Chayote with Tropical Fruit
SERVES: 4

Chef Pat Vanderberg created this colorful dish. The dressing is delicious, and can be used with other salads, or as a marinade for fish, or grilled chicken.

Ingredients:

4 4-oz. chicken breasts, boneless,
  skinless and sliced into strips
1 tsp. lemongrass
salt and ground pepper to taste
Pam vegetable spray
4 c. romaine, spinach, and other deep
  green veggies
½ c. strawberries, halved
1 c. blueberries or blackberries, fresh
  or frozen, unsweetened
1 c. chayote, diced
½ persimmon, very ripe, chopped
1 celery stalk, diced small

Dressing:
1 c. raspberries, fresh or frozen
  unsweetened
½ tsp. orange rind, grated
¼ c. orange juice
1 tsp. lemon rind, grated
1 tbsp. key lime juice
1 tbsp. fresh mint, chopped
1 tsp. honey
¼ tsp. salt

Method:
1. Season chicken with lemongrass, salt and pepper.
2. Spray pan with Pam and pan fry chicken until all the pink is gone. Keep warm.
3. Arrange greens on 4 large white plates.
4. Decorate with fruits, chayote, persimmon, and celery.
5. Evenly divide strips of chicken over top of each salad. Set aside.

Dressing:
1. In food processor or blender, puree raspberries.
2. Add orange rind and juice, lemon rind and juice, mint, honey, and salt. Process until well blended. Shake well before serving.
3. Dribble salads with dressing or serve on side in small dressing or sauce dish.
4. Garnish salads with ½ c. mandarin oranges
5. Serve.

Tropical Diet Food Servings
Plain salad, no dressing: 2 protein, 1 fruit
With dressing: 2 protein, 2 fruit

Mahi Tropical
SERVES: 2

A fish similar to flounder, popular in Miami and the tropics.

Ingredients:

1 tsp. lemon pepper
2 oz. garlic cloves
Pam vegetable cooking spray
¼ c. yellow bell pepper, chopped
⅛ c. red bell pepper, chopped
⅛ c. green bell pepper, chopped

2 4-oz. pieces Mahi Mahi fish
kosher salt and fresh ground black
   peppers to taste

Garnish:
Fresh Parsley

Method:

1. Marinate mahi mahi with lemon pepper. Set aside.
2. Sauté garlic cloves in Pam sprayed large frying pan until slightly brown.
3. Add peppers, and spray pan and peppers with Pam.
4. Continuing sautéing at low heat until all vegetables are slightly brown and wilted, but still bright. Set aside.
5. Spray pan with Pam, and place Mahi Mahi pieces. Fry on both sides at high heat until seared.
6. Add vegetables to top, or put vegetables on each plate first, and place fish on top. Season with fresh pepper and salt.
7. Garnish with fresh parsley.

Chef Michelle's Tips

Mahi Mahi can be substituted with any white fish, such as snapper, pompano, or sole.

Tropical Diet Food Servings: 3 protein, 1 cup veggies

Tropical Brownies

SERVES 12

This ready-to-make, fat free brownie mix is a big hit with family and friends. They won't know the brownies are nonfat if you don't tell them! Delicious and nutritious with any tropical fruit.

Ingredients:

1 No Pudge Brownie mix
⅔ c. nonfat vanilla yogurt
Pam vegetable cooking spray
¼ c. tropical fruit, diced small

Fruit possibilities, your choice:
kiwi
persimmon
quince
papaya
chayote (technically a veggie)
berries-fresh, or frozen unsweetened
apple
pear
raisins

Method:

1. Preheat oven to 350° F.
2. Blend nonfat yogurt with No Pudge in a large glass bowl. If the mix is thick, don't worry. You can add a tablespoon or more of yogurt to make the mixing easier.
3. Add ¼ cup tropical fruit, your choice and mix throughout.
4. Spoon mixture into 8 x 8 in. pan sprayed with Pam vegetable spray.
5. Bake for 32 to 34 minutes. Let cool, cut, and enjoy with no guilt!

⏀ Nutrition Nugget

The fruit adds extra fiber, gives the brownie dimension, provides you with a greater feeling of fullness. The fruits have oodles of additional vitamins and minerals.

Tropical Diet Food Servings: 1½ starch, ½ fruit

Tuna Tartar on Plantain Wafer

SERVES 4

Great for family or company designed by Chef Michelle.

Ingredients:

¼ lb. tuna, fresh, sliced
2 tsp. chili oil
¼ c. cilantro, chopped
¼ c. chopped chives
1 oz. red onion, chopped

1 tbsp. ginger, peeled and grated
½ plantain, green, boiled, mashed
sea salt and black pepper for taste
Pam vegetable spray
1 tsp. sesame oil-drizzle for top

Method

1. Preheat oven to 350° F.
2. Combine tuna with seasoning. Mix well.
3. Set aside in refrigerator, until ready to serve.
4. Take boiled and mashed plantain. Season with sea salt and black pepper.
5. Divide into four "patties" and bake on Pam sprayed baking sheet for about 15 minutes, until browned.
6. Remove and let cool.
7. Top each patty with tuna mix, and drizzle with sesame oil.
8. Ready to serve.

Tropical Diet Food Servings: 1 protein, 1 fat, ½ starch

A La Vodka Caribbean Style
Chef Michelle Austin
SERVES: 6 TO 8

A delicious sauce that works well over shrimp, chicken, pasta, brown rice, or most veggie dishes.

Ingredients:

Pam olive oil cooking spray
3 garlic cloves, minced
2 onions, chopped
10 tomatoes, fresh, peeled, and
  chopped
1 hot pepper, Scotch Bonnet*
1 green pepper
1 red pepper
1 small can of tomato paste
½ c. lite whipping cream

½ tsp. sea salt
½ tsp. cumin
1 tsp. sugar (could also use Splenda)
4 oz. *Imperia*™ vodka, or to taste

choose the heat level you desire

Optional:
Black pepper
Cilantro, fresh, chopped to taste

Method:

1. Heat Pam in medium to high heated large pan.
2. Sauté onions and garlic for 2 minutes, or until translucent.
3. Add tomatoes, sauté for another minute.
4. Add tomato paste, whipping cream, and sugar.
5. Reduce heat, and simmer with lid on for 15 minutes at medium to low temperature.
6. Add spices, and vodka little-by-little to suit your taste. *Use any leftover vodka for a quick shot before dinnertime!*
7. Cook an additional 5 to 10 minutes.
8. Remove from heat and serve over your favorite shrimp, chicken, pasta, or brown rice dish.

Tropical Diet Food Servings
For 6 servings: 1 cups veggies, 3 fats
For 8 servings: 1 cup veggies, 1½ fats

Key Lime Vodka Martini
SERVES: 2

While vodka is not your typical island beverage, it may prevent some of the hangovers you may experience after drinking other alcoholic beverages—especially after spending a night-on-the-town, partying and dancing in Caribbean style.

Ingredients:

2 oz. vodka

Juice from 4 key limes

2 oz. contreau

Sugar-simple syrup

Method:
1. Mix ingredients with crushed ice in martini shaker.
2. Taste for sweetness and adjust as needed.
3. Garnish glass with sugar and key lime wheel.

 Nutrition Nugget ————————————————————

A vitamin A-, C-, and potassium-rich, island drink. ——————————

Bahama Mama
A la Chef Michelle

Ingredients:

1 *Imperia*™ vodka shot
2 oz. Tropicana® fortified orange juice
1½ oz. coconut milk

1½ oz. unsweetened pineapple juice
1 grenadine splash

Method:

1. Mix ingredients with crushed ice in martini shaker.
2. Top off with grenadine.

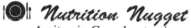 *Nutrition Nugget*

A vitamin C, and potassium-rich party drink. You get less fat per serving, when you use lite coconut milk.

Tropical Diet Food Servings: 1 fruit, 1 fat

Cooking Essentials: It's Measurable

So how do you prepare all the delicious recipes we have in store for you in Chapter 9.

Now that you have your staple and substitution lists, your seasoning guide and portion cheat sheet, here's how to measure up in the kitchen whether you're following an English recipe or converting to metric.

This	is equal to:
Dash	less than 1/8th teaspoon
3 tsp.	1 tbsp.
2 tbsp.	1oz
4 tbsp.	¼ cup
5⅓ tbsp.	⅓ cup
8 tbsp.	½ cup
1 cup	½ pint
2 cups	1 pint
4 cups	1 quart
2 pints	1 quart
4 quarts	1 gallon

CONVERSION TO METRIC

To convert from	To	Multiply by
Teaspoons (tsp.)	milliliters (ml)	5
Tablespoons (Tbsp.)	milliliters (ml)	15
Fluid ounces (fl. oz.)	milliliters (ml)	30
Cups (c)	liters (l)	.24
Pints (pt)	liters (l)	.47
Quarts (qt)	liters (l)	.95

AND BACK AGAIN

Milliliters (ml)	fluid ounces (fl. oz)	.03
Liters (l)	pints (pt)	2.1
	quarts (qt.)	1.06
	gallons (gal)	.26

Simply a substitution

This is the ingredient substitution list which shows you what to use when you're in a jam. While there is no nutritional savings in this category of ingredient substitutions, this list will help you when the cupboard is dry. Trust me, we all run out of ingredients at some point in our cooking careers.

Ingredient and purpose	Substitution
1 cup heavy cream	⅔ cup milk and ⅓ cup butter
1 teaspoon baking powder	1 tsp. baking soda and 1 tsp. cream of tartar or ¼ tsp. baking soda and ½ c buttermilk—reduce other recipe liquids by ½
1 cup mini-marshmallows	10 large marshmallows
1 cup sugar	1 cup honey—reduce liquids in recipe by ¼ cup, reduce baking temperature by 25° F
1 garlic clove	⅛ tsp. garlic powder or ¼ tsp. garlic salt (reduce salt by ⅛ tsp.)
1 tbsp. fresh herbs	1 tsp. dried herbs or ¼ tsp. powdered herbs or ¼ tsp. herb salt (reduce salt ¼ tsp.)

1 medium onion (2½" diameter)	2 tbsp. instant minced onion or 1 tsp. onion powder or 2 tsp. onion salt (reduce salt by 1 tsp.)
1 cup buttermilk	1 tbsp. lemon juice or vinegar and enough regular milk to make 1 cup
1 cup heavy whipped cream	⅔ cup well-chilled evaporated nonfat milk, whipped
1 square chocolate	3 tbsp. cocoa and 1 tbsp. butter or butter sub equivalent
1 cup all purpose flour	1 cup plus 2 tbsp. cake flour
1 cup cake flour	1 cup minus 2 tbsp. all-purpose flour
1 tbsp. cornstarch	2 tbsp. flour or 1½ tbsp. quick cooking tapioca

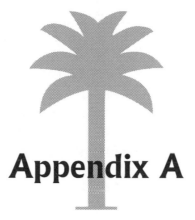

Appendix A

Tropical Food Glossary

Ackee

Name: *Ackee*

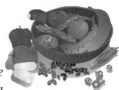

Introduced to Jamaica from West Africa during the slave trade in 1787. This is also known as Jamaica poisoning because if ackee is eaten before ripening, it's poisonous. Ackee and salt fish is a Jamaica national staple.

What does it look like? Bell-pepper shaped, reddish-yellow. When ripe, it bursts open to display shiny black seeds covered by a creamy, yellow flesh, which is the edible portion.

Taste: Fresh ackee has lemony flavor.

Texture: Fresh has a similar texture to scrambled eggs firm, and oily aril surrounds shiny, black seeds.

Purchasing: Immature and overmature fruits are poisonous. Can be purchased canned by Grace Company.

Storage: In United States, primarily found in can.

Serving Tips: Traditionally, served with saltfish, but can also go with shellfish or vegetables. Can be mixed into scrambled eggs for those needing additional dietary calories.

Nutrition Facts: ($3^1{}_2$ oz. canned)

Tropical Diet servings: 1 fruit, 2 fats
   140 calories, 11 grams carbohydrates, 4 grams protein, 9 grams fat, 3.5 grams saturated fat, 125 mg sodium, 2 grams fiber.

Vitamins/Minerals: Vitamin A and C, calcium, iron, phosphorus, and niacin.

Avocado

Name: *Avocado*

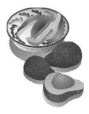

Native to Central America discovered in 1526. Known as the alligator pear and testicle fruit since it had a reputation as an aphrodisiac. Cultivated in Florida, and California. Remained unknown to Europeans until after World War II. The largest producers are Mexico, the United States, Dominican Republic, Brazil, and Columbia.

What does it look like? A round to pear-shaped, green, shiny skinned fruit.

Taste: Nutty.

Texture: Creamy with a huge pit.

Purchasing and Storage: Choose heavy-for-size avocados, free of black spots and bruises. Ripen at room temperature. Can accelerate ripening process by placing in paper bag. Avocados will not continue to ripen after refrigeration.

Serving ideas: Raw, salads, fruit salads, guacamole, and sandwiches.

Nutrition Facts: ($\frac{1}{2}$ medium)
161 calories, 7 grams carbohydrates, 2 grams protein, 15 grams fat, 5 grams fiber.

Vitamins/Minerals: Excellent potassium and folic acid source. Good in B_6. Also contains copper, Vitamins A, C, B1, B3, iron, and zinc.

Phytochemicals: More lutein than any other fruit. Also contains glutathione and phytoesterol which inhibit cholesterol production.

Health benefits: Good source of healthy fats; may be good for stomach, intestines and digestion; avocado oil used in cosmetics.

🍽 *Nutrition Nugget*

Florida avocados have fewer calories and fat than California avocados. Florida 110 calories and 9 grams fat. California 175 calories and 17 grams fat per $3\frac{1}{2}$ oz serving.

Banana

Name: *Banana*

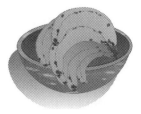

According to Indian legend, the banana was the fruit offered to Adam. This is why it is called the fruit of paradise. Originally from Indo-Malaysian region, 4,000 years ago. The banana was not introduced to the Americas until the Philadelphia Centennial Exhibition of the 1800s. The leading selling fruit in the United States, second leading crop in the world. Some of the most important export crops in the Caribbean are bananas, although India is the largest banana grower. Plantains, the green, cooking banana are a staple in many parts of the world.

What does it look like? Elongated, 5 to 10 inch, curved, tropical fruit with a smooth outer skin that peels easily when the fruit is ripe. Latin American red bananas are slightly wider and heavier. Manzano, a.k.a., finger or apple bananas are short and chubby with a mild strawberry apple flavor. (Bananas turn fully black when ripe). Cooking or green plantains are green to yellow, brown to black.

Taste: Bananas become sweeter as they ripen. When unripe plantains are cooked, they have no banana flavor.

Texture: Smooth

Purchasing: Buy slightly lustrous peel with some small brown specs.

Storage: Unripe bananas should not be refrigerated, ripe can be stored in refrigerator up to 2 weeks;

Serving Tips: Fresh out the skin; sliced on cereal, in yogurt, frozen desserts, chopped in muffin and cake mixes; (frozen peel off the skin first), saut ed or fried with cinnamon and ginger sprinkled on top.

Nutrition Facts: 1 medium banana
109 calories, 28 grams carbohydrates, 1 gram protein, and fat, 3 grams fiber.

Vitamins/Minerals: Great source of B6 and potassium. Good source of vitamin C. Also, have magnesium, phosphorus, vitamin A, and folic acid. Red bananas and plantains are a good source of vitamin A.

Black Sapote

Name: *Black Sapote*

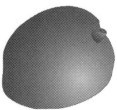

Native to Mexico cultivated prior to the 1600s. Known as the chocolate fruit. Same family as persimmon, a.k.a. black persimmon. Cultivated in Florida, the Philippines, Dominican Republic, and Cuba.

What does it look like? Tomato-like fruit 10 to 13 cm diameter. Varies in size, softball to another half size up. Thin and firm, shiny green rind with brown specs covers rich, dark brown colored, custard like flesh.

Taste: Must eat ripened for sweet, nut-like flavor. Great chocolate substitute. Flavor enhanced by vanilla or rum.

Texture: Black, creamy custard like pulp.

Purchasing: Firm, bruise-free, olive-green skin, ripe fruit feels like a marshmallow in the hand.

Storage: Fruit does not change color as it matures. However, can be hard one day, soft the next. Store at room temperature, uncovered, out of direct sun until ripe. Then refrigerate unwashed in plastic or paper bag. Will keep 3 to 5 days. Pulp can be frozen in moisture proof sealed container for 2 to 3 months.

Serving Tips: Great, low cal, chocolate substitute. Fresh out of rind, can be frozen, or used in bread, muffin, or cake recipes.

Nutrition Facts: 3½ oz. pulp
134 calories, 34 grams carbohydrates, 2 grams protein, 0 fat.

Vitamins/Minerals: Rich in vitamins A and C, and potassium. Also have niacin, iron, phosphorus, and calcium.

📖 CHRIS NOTES:
Known as the chocolate pudding fruit, but does not taste like chocolate. Sweet taste, not distinctive. Used in brownie, ice cream, and desserts. Mixed with Cool Whip®, makes a great ice cream.

Callaloo

Name: *Callaloo*

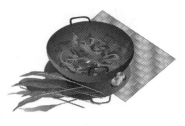

A.k.a., bhaji, the main ingredient in a hearty soup. Can be used in place of spinach in vegetable dishes, stews, pasta plates, and as a side dish to increase dietary calcium.

What does it look like? A bushy, light-green vegetable, with thin-veined leaves very similar to spinach and kale. Tin a.k.a. canned variety has washed-out-green look, but similar nutritional properties as fresh variety.

Taste: Similar to a green leafy vegetable. Easier to find canned in the U.S., imported from Jamaica.

Texture: Crunchy, like spinach leaves. Stringy and somewhat mushy in tin.

Purchasing: Canned from Jamaica Country Style Brand (JCI).

Storage: Canned storage suggest 3-month limit.

Serving Tips: Delicious addition to stews and soups, rice, couscous, vegetarian sides, or main courses.

Nutrition Facts: ½ cup
30 calories, 4 grams carbohydrates, 2 grams protein, 0 fat, 1 gram fiber.

Vitamins/Minerals: Vitamin A, iron, calcium.

Health benefits: Excellent source of vitamin A and calcium, moderate source of iron.

📖 CHRIS NOTES:

In Jamaica, comes from amaranth leaves. In Trinidad, comes from taro leaves.

Carambola

Name: *Carambola*

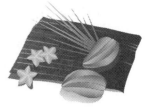

A.k.a., starfruit, because the fruit has 4 to 6 vertical lobes that result in a star shape when cut crosswise. In Portuguese, means fruit appetizer. A native of Malaysia, cultivated in Southeast Asia for many centuries, introduced to Florida in 1887, and later Hawaii. Major suppliers include Taiwan, Malaysia, Guyana, India, the Philippines, Australia, and Israel.

What does it look like? A 2 to 6-inch oval-to-elliptical, 3 oz. to 4 oz. greenish-yellow fruit, with a thin, shiny, edible, waxy skin, light to dark yellow flesh and up to 12 small edible seeds enclosed by a thin, gelatinous pocket.

Taste: There are two major types tart and sweet.

Texture: Crunchy and juicy.

Purchasing: Easily damaged, best to choose fruits that are firm, and shiny with a sweet fruity aroma.

Storage: Can refrigerate for about 3 weeks without damage or loss in food quality. Fruits which are picked before fully ripe will turn yellow at room temperature.

Serving Tips: Before serving, remove ridge of cells and cut the fruit crosswise. Sweet, eaten fresh whole or sliced. Great garnish for meat, poultry, and fish dishes, sliced and cooked in stir-fry, or fresh in vegetable and fruit salads. Puree for chutneys, salsas. Makes a good juice and can replace mangos in chutney.

Nutrition Facts: 1 fruit
42 calories, 10 grams carbohydrates, 1 gram protein, 0 fat, 3 grams fiber.

Vitamins/Minerals: Excellent source of vitamin C. Good source of vitamin A. Also has potassium, magnesium, phosphorus, and folic acid.

Health benefits: Low-calorie, low-sugar, fruit with a good amount of fiber.

📖 CHRIS NOTES:

Misunderstood fruit. Can utilize when green and make a fried, green tomato-type dish. Also good as a relish, jelly, and pickled. Also contains oxalic acid which may precipitate kidney stones if eaten in very large amounts.

Chayote

Name: *Chayote*

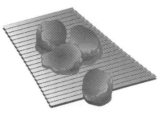

A.k.a. christophene, cho-cho, mango-squash, and choke. Cultivated by Aztecs and Mayans long before Columbus arrived—the name is derived by the Mayan word chayotli. A tropical member of the cucumber and squash family is actually a fruit. In Louisiana, called mirliton, in Florida a vegetable pear. Native to Mexico, Central America, and West Indies.

What does it look like? A white or mint-green, pear. Shape resembles avocado or summer squash. Has a ridged, prickly skin. Can vary in size and color.

Taste: Can vary in texture and flavor. Takes on tastes of seasoning.

Texture: Cucumber-like, crunchy, juicy texture.

Purchasing: Choose firm, unblemished, clear green. Available year-round. Peak season is late summer through early fall.

Storage: Up to 1-month, uncovered in cool, dry, dark place or in a perforated plastic bag in refrigerator. Also can be stored in vegetable crisper for up to one week.

Serving Tips: Easily prepared by steaming with or without skin. The skin remains firm. Great for stuffing. The flesh becomes transparent after cooking. It takes on colors of spices or other foods. Raw, diced, and added to salad, chutney, or guacamole. Serve as crudit s and dip instead of cucumbers. Stuff for main or side dish. Also can be used in soups, stews, even brownies (see Tropical Brownie recipe on page 217). Great substitute for carrots and zucchini in breads and pastries. Can also be made into applesauce, chutney, or apple type strudel.

Nutrition Facts: $\frac{1}{2}$ cup
17 calories, 4 grams carbohydrate, 1 gram protein, 0 fat, 2 grams fiber.

Vitamins/Minerals: Great source of vitamin C and potassium. Also includes calcium, vitamin A, folic acid, phosphorus, and magnesium.

◉ *Nutrition Nugget*

Wear gloves when preparing chayote since it secretes a sticky substance during peeling which can dry out your hands.

📖 CHRIS NOTES:

Fresh is best. Use caution when preparing fruit without gloves, hands get coated and flaky. Also, cook for short amounts of time, otherwise becomes grey and mushy.

Cassava

Name: *Cassava or Yuca*

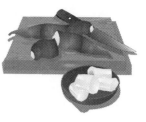

A root vegetable, originally cultivated by Arawak Indians. Introduced to Africa and Far East, from Brazil, Paraguay, and the Caribbean. Staple food in many African countries, Asia, Central, and South America. In some countries goes by the name yuca. Nigeria, Brazil, Thailand, Zaire, and Indonesia are the world's leading producers.

What does it look like? When it s small, it looks like sweet potato.

Taste: Bland which absorbs the flavors of other foods. Two varieties, sweet and bitter. Bitter is poisonous. Cannot be eaten raw.

Texture: Similar to potato.

Purchasing: Buy with no signs of mold or sticky patches, as little damage as possible. Avoid acrid or sour-smelling tubers with grey blue mottling.

Storage: Spoils easily and is damaged by exposure to high humidity, and high temperatures above 68… F. Extremely perishable, does not hold up to shipping. Refrigerate no more than 4 days. Can also be cut into pieces and frozen.

Serving Tips: Before cooking, rinse the cassava well. Boil keeping the pot lid on the saucepan. Peeled cassava is served mashed or boiled, baked, sliced, and pan fried. Peeled root can also be grated and the starch extracted to make bread, crackers, pasta, and tapioca pearls (commercial). Sweet cassava can be baked and served like a potato which is interchangeable in most recipes. Delicious addition to stews and soup. Tapioca, the starch obtained in commercial processing, forms whitish beads of varying sizes. Can also be processed into flake, flour, or granular forms for instant tapioca. Takes only 10 minutes to prepare.

Nutrition Facts: $\frac{1}{4}$ cup
83 calories, 20 grams carbohydrate, 1 gram protein, less than 1 gram fat and fiber.

Vitamins/Minerals: Vitamin C, potassium, iron, magnesium, and a good source of B1. Also contains folic acid, phosphorus, and pantothenic acid.

Cherimoya

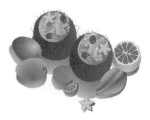

Name: *Cherimoya*

A.k.a., custard apple, the name derived from chirmoya means cold seed in Quenchua, the Inca language still spoken by the Inca people of Peru and Bolivia. Over 50 varieties most developed in California. Belongs to the custard-apple family which includes soursop and sweetsop.

What does it look like? Bronze to green, turning yellow and black as fruit ripens depending on variety. Oval, spherical, or heart shaped, weighing between $^1{}_2$ and $4^1{}_2$ pounds. Some varieties covered with fingerprint like markings and large overlapping lobes.

Taste: Pulp is sweet and juicy with slightly acidic taste. Like a blend of papaya, pineapple, and banana.

Texture: Inedible skin covers fragrant whitish pulp, granular texture. Consistency of custard. Contains numerous hard and inedible seeds.

Purchasing: Usually picked before it s ripe, since it does not travel nor store well.

Storage: Cherimoyas are very fragile and should be stored in the refrigerator for no more than 2 days.

Serving Tips: Served raw, scooped, and eaten with a spoon. Sprinkle with orange juice to prevent discoloration if adding to salads or dishes. Left at room temperature, pulp can be pureed and added to sorbets, yogurt, ice cream, smoothies, cake, muffin, and pastry mixes. Fruit itself can be served frozen and eaten like an ice cream.

Nutrition Facts: ⅛ fruit
64 calories, 16 grams carbohydrate, 1 gram protein, 0 fat, 2 grams fiber.

Vitamins/Minerals: Vitamin C, calcium, and phosphorus.

📖 CHRIS NOTES:
Seeds are toxic. Do not use in blended smoothies. Remove seeds before consumption.

Chili

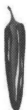

Name: *Chili*

One of the first plants to be cultivated in South America more than 7,000 years ago. Member of the nightshade family which includes the eggplant, potato, tamarillo, tomato, and alkekengi. Unknown to Europe until Christopher Columbus brought them in 1492. From there, they spread around the world. Over 150 varieties in Mexico alone.

Taste: The heat level is determined by the capsaicin it contains, the compound concentrated in the ribs and seeds. Chilies pickled or raw have more heat than cooked chilies. The heat level is measured in Scoville units on a scale of 0 to 300,000. The hottest chile is the habanero. The heat level will vary depending on where it was grown, when it was picked, the irrigation, the weather, and the growing season, so Scoville units are only a guide. The ratings have been simplified to 1 to 10 to make them easier to remember.

The following are the most commonly used fresh chilies.

¥ **Habanero-dried:** level 10. It s so hot that even when pureed the fumes from the blender can scorch the skin. Used to make bottled hot chili sauces.

¥ **Serrano:** Level 8. Small chili, $1\frac{1}{2}$-2 inches long with a pointed tip. Used in cooked dishes, guacamole, and salsas.

¥ **Fresno:** Level 8. Look like long elongated sweet peppers, $2\frac{1}{2}$ inches long and $\frac{3}{4}$ inch wide. Hot, sweet flavor used in salsas, meat, fish, and vegetables dishes.

¥ **Jalapeno:** Level 6. Most common and popular. The same length as the Serrano, but plumper. Sold at all stages of ripeness, likely to find them in red or green. Green are often pickled. Typically stuffed with cheese, coated in batter and deep fried for an appetizer.

¥ **Pablano:** Level 3. Large chilies, $3\frac{1}{2}$ inches long and $2\frac{1}{4}$ inches wide and sometimes heart shaped. Has a rich, earthy flavor which is intensified with cooking.

Purchasing: Look for firm, fresh chilies with brightly colored shiny skin. Avoid limp or dull chilies.

Storage: Store in a plastic bag unwashed in the refrigerator for up to one week.

Nutrition Facts: 100 grams
40 calories, 9.6 grams carbohydrates, 2 grams protein, 0 fat and 1.8 grams fiber.

Vitamins/Minerals: Higher vitamin C content than oranges, however since they are used in small amounts. Most won t get the dose.

Health benefits: Capsaicin is an alkaloid which stimulates salivation and causes gastric juices to flow. For some, this aids digestion.

Chef's Tips
Always use gloves when cutting and preparing chilies to avoid deep heat and pain from the capsaicin. Also, if you bite into a chili that is uncomfortably hot, swallow a teaspoon of sugar. Drinking water will only spread the heat further.

CHRIS NOTES:
Caution wear gloves when preparing chilis to avoid getting *burned*!

Dasheen

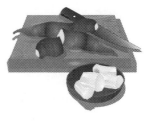

Name: *Dasheen*

A.k.a. taro, a starchy vegetable which is toxic if eaten raw. More than 500 varieties from around the world. One of the oldest plants, important part of Asian diet and rituals. In 2,000 B.C., taro was brought from S.E. Asia to the Pacific Rim and N.E. Asia. Brought to Hawaii in 400 to 500 A.D. by the first Tahitian, and Marquesan settlers. Staple in the diets of West Africa, Caribbean, and Polynesian islands.

Taste: Cooked has somewhat nutty flavor similar to potatoes or water chestnuts.

Texture: Like a potato, gray white to lilac flesh.

Purchasing: firm with no sign of mold or soft patches.

Storage: Cool, dry location.

Serving Tips: Must be cooked thoroughly to neutralize the toxic calcium oxalate crystals they contain. Peeled and cooked like potatoes.

Nutrition Facts: ½ cup cooked root
94 calories, 23 grams carbohydrates, no protein or fat.

½ cup cooked leaves 17 calories, 3 grams carbohydrates, 2 grams protein, and 0 fats.

Vitamins/Minerals: B6 and potassium. Taro leaves are high in vitamin A, and C, potassium, folate and calcium.

📖 CHRIS NOTES:
If raw, leaves can be highly irritating. Eat cooked leaves only.

Ginger

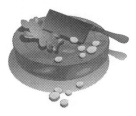

Name: *Ginger*

Native to Southeast Asia cultivated in tropical countries. Mentioned in ancient Chinese and Indian writings. Was also known to the Greeks.

What does it look like? Like arthritic fingers with a root skin.

Taste: Highly aromatic and pungent, pulp can be very hot.

Texture: Fibrous dry stem, with a thin, edible skin, varying in color from sandy to white, and red.

Purchasing: Available fresh, dried and preserved. Choose fresh, firm and smooth, free of mold with a uniform buff color.

Storage: Fresh in refrigerator for 2 to 3 weeks in a plastic bag. Peel just before using. Can be frozen as is. Candied keeps indefinitely. Preserved should be refrigerated once the jar is open.

Serving Tips: Peeled sliced, grated, minced or julienne; added to vegetable, rice, couscous, fruit and vegetable salads, desserts, meats, stir-fry almost any baked product.

Nutrition Facts: 3 tbsp.
40 calories, 9 grams carbohydrates, 1 gram protein, 1 gram fat.

Vitamins/Minerals: Rich in potassium, also has magnesium and phosphorus.

Health benefits: Aromatic and medicinal properties as a tonic, antiseptic, diuretic, aphrodisiac, and fever reducer. Aids the appetite. Also stimulates digestion and combats gas. Effective against colds, coughs, car sickness, and rheumatic pain.

Guava

Name: *Guava*

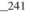
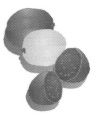

A.k.a. guyava, originally cultivated by Incas, grown in Africa, Australia, India, Brazil, Taiwan, and the southern U.S. Native to southern Mexico. Member of the myrtle family of cinnamon, nutmeg, clove, eucalyptus, and feijoa.

What does it look like? A small, round or oval, golf-ball size fruit with a pale yellow, wrinkled skin, covering a variety of flesh which can vary depending on variety from white, yellow, or salmon. Skin covers 100 to 500 tiny, peach-colored edible seed-laden, soft pulp.

Taste: Fragrant, slightly acidic taste. Like a combination of a pear and a strawberry.

Texture: Firm and mealy.

Purchasing: Smooth, unblemished fruits which are neither too hard nor too soft.

Storage: Ripen at room temperature in 1 to 5 days. Place in paper bag to accelerate ripening process. Refrigerate in perforated plastic bag to slow down ripening. Mature green can be kept for several weeks. Can be frozen for extended periods of time. Fruit which has changed color should be eaten in a few days because it will bruise easily and rot.

Serving Tips: Perfect fresh, sliced for snacking, pureed for smoothies, bread, and muffin mixes, chopped for breads, pancakes, or as coulis for desserts. Also, warm topping for pancakes and/or main course dishes. Found commercially as juice, nectar, and as a popular Latin paste to spread on bread. In Mexico, guava and sweet potato is a favorite combination.

Nutrition Facts: 1 guava, no seed
46 calories, 11 grams carbohydrates, 1 gram protein, 1 gram fat, 5 grams fiber.

Vitamins/Minerals: Good source of vitamin A (beta-carotene) and C. Health benefits: Great low-calorie snack for dieters, high-carbohydrate, low-fat food for athletes. Chock-full-of vitamin A, C and lycopene which all act as anti-oxidants. Also known for astringent and laxative properties.

📖 **CHRIS NOTES:**

Missed opportunity in the food world. Cooked or fresh delicious. One of the most popular fruits in the Latin community.

Jackfruit

Name: *Jackfruit*

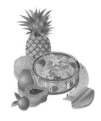

Indigenous to the rainforests of India, native to the region between India and Malaysia. It's the largest tree-borne fruit in the world, reaching 80 pounds, 36 inches and 20 inches in diameter. Relative of breadfruit.

What does it look like? Oval, pale green to dark yellow rind covered with short, sharp, hexagonal, fleshy spine. The flesh has soft, yellow bulbs, enclosing hundreds of smooth oval, light brown seeds.

Taste: Two types, one is sweet like banana, and fleshy. The other is crisp and crunchy with a less sweet flavor.

Texture: Fibrous, soft with texture like oysters.

Purchasing: After ripening, the fruit turns brown and spoils very quickly. Choose fruits without bruises or soft spots. Can buy canned from JCS.

Storage: Will keep at room temperature for 3 to 10 days. Cut or ripe should be refrigerated.

Serving Tips: When cutting, wear disposable gloves so fingers do not become sticky with the juice. Eaten as a vegetable when it is unripe, as a fruit when ripe. Boil, fry, roast, or freeze. Preserved to be dried, or canned. Seeds boiled, or roasted, and eaten like chestnuts. In India, used in curries. Can also be preserved by drying or canning.

Nutrition Facts: ½ cup
78 calories, 121 % water, 1 gram fiber and protein, 20 grams carbohydrates.

JCS brand canned 4 pieces, 130 calories, 34 grams carbohydrates, 28 grams sugar, 1 gram fiber,

Vitamins/Minerals: Vitamins C, A, potassium, magnesium, and calcium.

Health benefits: Fresh and healthy, low-fat, sweet alternative to cakes, cookies, and candy. Especially good frozen as a snack, or added to low-fat brownie, or muffin mix for texture.

📖 **CHRIS NOTES:**
Fantastic fresh, in salads. Also for ice cream, and even frozen as snack.

Jicama

Name: *Jicama*

Native to Mexico, Central, and South America, a.k.a., yam bean, to the Aztecs who used the seeds as medicine. In the 17th century, the Spanish explorers brought the plant to the Philippines, where cultivation throughout Asia and the pacific spread quickly.

What does it look like? Slight squat shape, looks like a turnip with slightly flattened ends, and a thin, brown, inedible skin which covers a juicy white flesh.

Taste: Juicy and slightly sweet.

Texture: Juicy flesh, crunchy like a water chestnut.

Purchasing: Ready-to-eat at any stage of growth. Choose a firm, medium-size, or small with thin skin. Large, thick-skinned tend to be fibrous and dry.

Storage: Unwrapped in the refrigerator for 3 weeks, stored like potatoes in a cool, dry place for several weeks. Once cut, will store for about a week refrigerated.

Serving Tips: Fresh sprinkled with lemon, or key lime juice, and seasoned with chili powder. Raw sliced julienne, sliced or cubed and served with dip or guacamole. Cooked remains crunchy. Perfect for soup, stews, rice, vegetable, quiches, tofu, meat, poultry, seafood, and fruit salads. Jicama absorbs flavor without losing texture. Can replace water chestnuts and bamboo shoots in most recipes.

Nutrition Facts: ½ cup
23 calories, 5 grams carbohydrates, 1 gram protein and 0 grams fat, 3 grams fiber.

Vitamins/Minerals: Good source of vitamin C also has potassium and phosphorus.

Health benefits: Low-calorie, high-fiber vegetable, ideal for filling dieters with a great tortilla chip alternative to serve with guacamole dip.

Key Lime

Name: *Key lime*

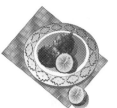

Product of South Florida and Latin America. Brooks Tropicals in Homestead Florida is one of the only commercial growers that sell key limes beyond the state line. Lime trees themselves date back to the 13th century when they were brought to France and Italy by the crusaders. Christopher Columbus brought the lime seeds to Hispaniola on his trip to the new world in 1493.

What does it look like? Thin, tight skin covers a fragrant juicy pulp.

Taste: Flavor is a little bit more limey than tart.

Texture: Juicy, fibrous pulp.

Purchasing: Fresh off a local Florida tree or out of the bottle from the Key West Lime Juice Factory. If fresh, choose firm and heavy for size. Avoid dull-colored, soft, or dried out fruits.

Storage: More perishable than lemons, needs handling care. Left at room temperature will last about a week. Can be stored up to 10 days in a plastic bag placed in refrigerator. Juice and zest can be frozen.

Serving Tips: to get the maximum juice out of the key lime, roll it back and forth a few times, pressing down as though massaging it before cutting.* Use as a tenderizer and flavor enhancer for meats and poultry; in beverages such as the tropical margarita and in the classic key lime pie

Nutrition Facts: 1 lime
20 calories, 7 grams carbohydrates, O protein and fat, 2 grams fiber.

Vitamins/Minerals: High in vitamin C also has potassium, and calcium.

📖 CHRIS NOTES:
This is the real lime, all others are hybrids of the lime fruit. Any lime can be substituted for the key lime.

*Tip from Donna Shields, author of Caribbean Light Cookbook.

Kiwi

Name: *Kiwi*

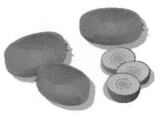

The most nutritionally dense fruit. Once considered a delicacy, called yang tao by the great khans of China, who relished the fruit's brilliant color. Introduced to New Zealand in 1906, brown fuzzy, emerald green fleshed fruit; named after a bird it resembled. A.k.a. strawberry peach or Chinese gooseberry in English.

What does it look like? A fuzzy, brown, golf ball.

Taste: Cross between banana, strawberry, and papaya.

Texture: Soft and creamy except for miniature black edible seeds.

Purchasing: Firm and unbruised.

Storage: Room temperature up to 7 days. Refrigerated up to 3 weeks.

Serving Tips: Sliced in cereal, yogurt, jams, chutney, frozen smoothies, daiquiris, and martinis. Garnish or just fresh.

Nutrition Facts: (140 g)
90 calories, 21 grams carbohydrates, 1 gram protein, 0 fat, 5 grams fiber.

Vitamins/Minerals: More potassium than a banana, twice the vitamin C of an orange, also folate, magnesium, vitamin E and copper.

Phytochemicals: Lutein which reduces the risk of cancer, heart disease, and macular degeneration.

Health benefits: Kiwi has been ranked the most nutritious fruit by some, followed by papaya, mango, and orange of the 27 most commonly eaten fruits.

📖 CHRIS NOTES:
Not tropical, sub-tropical. Was called the Chinese gooseberry until WW II, changed to kiwi by New Zealanders because of the political climate at the time.

Lychee

Name: *Lychee*

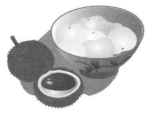

Also spelled litchi, originated in China more than 2,000 years ago. Tradition to offer as a good luck charm for the New Year. Considered a symbol of love. Nearly 75 varieties. Two most common in the U.S. are the Brewster and Mauritius. Prized by many as the most exquisite fruit.

What does it look like? 1 to 2 inches long, covered with an inedible, thin shell that is rough outside, and smooth inside. The shell hardens after the fruit is picked and is easy to remove. Inside is a translucent, pearly white flesh which encloses an inedible stone.

Taste: Fragrant and sweet, juicy flesh which combines the tastes of the strawberry, rose, and Muscat grape.

Texture: Flesh is crisp and juicy.

Purchasing: Sold fresh or canned in syrup which is most popular in U.S. Also dried or candied. Look for fruits with healthy blush, no cracks, with the stem attached.

Storage: Should be eaten at peak ripeness since unripe are gelatinous and overripe have no flavor. Placed in plastic bag and stored in refrigerator for 2 to 3 weeks, or in the freezer for up to 6 months.

Serving Tips: Eaten fresh in tropical countries, canned versions more common around U.S. Prepare fresh, sprinkled with key lime, lemon juice, or in berry combination in fruit salads. Stuffed with nonfat, cinnamon-seasoned cream cheese. Compliments meat, ham, chicken, or fish dishes.

Nutrition Facts: 10 fresh
63 calories, 81% water, 1 gram fiber and protein, 16 grams carbohydrates.

Vitamins/Minerals: Rich in vitamin C, good source of potassium. Also has phosphorus, and folic acid.

Mamey

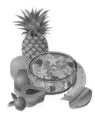

Name: *Mamey*

Native to the West Indies and Northern South America. Cultivated in Panama since the 1500s. Related to mangosteen. One of the largest and oldest fruiting plants has lived at Fairchild Tropical Gardens in Miami for more than 60 years.

What does it look like? A 4-inch to 8-inch, irregular round, heavy, and hard until ripe fruit. Light brown to grayish brown, inedible skin with rough, leathery texture which covers the apricot to red raspberry avocado textured flesh, and a single big inedible seed.

Taste: Could be sweet or bland depending on level of freshness.

Texture: Flesh is the texture of avocado flesh without all the fat.

Purchasing: Select hard fruit, free of blemish, not soft.

Storage: At room temperature, uncovered until ripe. Transfer to refrigerator for up to one week.

Serving Tips: Score skin from stem to apex. Remove in strips. Serve raw in slices as snack or in fruit salads. Add to pie and tarts, muffin, cake, and bread mixes for color, texture and flavor.

Nutrition Facts: about a ½ cup (3½ oz.)
51 calories, 13 grams carbohydrates, 0 grams protein and 0 grams fat, 3 grams fiber.

Vitamins/Minerals: Rich in vitamin C. Also contains vitamins A, B6, folic acid, iron, magnesium, copper, and calcium.

Health benefits: A low-calorie, vitamin and mineral-rich fruit with iron, and calcium and 3 grams of fiber. Ideal for female dieters and athletes.

📖 **CHRIS NOTES:**
An extremely popular Cuban fruit.

Mango

Name: *Mango*

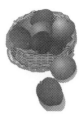

A native to India, sacred where it is the symbol of love. Cultivated for more than 6,000 years. Introduced to Brazil by the Portuguese. First appeared in Barbados in 1750. Same family as the cashew and pistachio. Most U.S. imports come from Mexico, while Puerto Rico, Florida, and California produces the rest of the crop.

What do they look like? Classified as a drupe, a fruit with a single seed, this 2 to 9 inch oval fruit has a smooth, inedible skin that varies from green to yellow to red. The yellow to orange flesh encloses a large fibrous seed.

Taste: Sweet and sour.

Texture: Soft, fibrous and juicy.

Purchasing: Choose neither too hard or too soft, without shriveled skin.

Storage: Partially ripe, will ripen at room temperature in about 3 to 5 days. Will ripen faster if placed in a paper bag. Ripe fruit will keep for 2 to 3 days in the refrigerator.

Serving Tips: Eat peeled, since the skin can be irritating to the mouth. Mango juice leaves indelible stains on clothing. Fresh, eaten as a snack, sliced or cubed for fruit and vegetable salads, pureed for cake, muffin, pancake, fruit toppings, blended with yogurt, used for smoothies, blended for coulis, as a side to meat or dessert dishes, or chopped for chutneys and salsas.

Nutrition Facts: $\frac{1}{2}$ raw
67 calories, 18 grams carbohydrates, 1 gram protein, 0 grams fat, 2 grams fiber.

Vitamins/Minerals: High in vitamin A (beta-carotene), and C. Also have potassium, phosphorus, calcium, and folic acid.

Phytochemicals: Rich in beta-carotene.

📖 CHRIS NOTES:
Best fruit in the world, however, when unripe, the fruit has a laxative effect. The skin can also cause an allergic reaction irritating the mouth and skin. Some people walk by a mango tree and have an allergic reaction.

Okra

Name: *Okra*

The godfather of vegetables, historians attribute introduction to Spain from Africa to Moorish invasions of Europe in the 8th century. Plant originated near Far East, and brought to North America and the Middle East in the 1700s by West African Slaves or the French colonists of Louisiana. Long considered a poor man's food and ignored by many, plant is a tropical sister of the cotton, hibiscus, and mallow family. The name is derived from the "Twi" word nkruman from the Gold Coast of Africa. A.k.a. lady fingers, gumbo and other regional names. Texas, Georgia, Florida, Alabama, and California are the leading producers.

What does it look like? Slightly curved, pale green, tapering hexagonal shaped 2 to 7 inch long pods have green fuzzy skin.

Taste: Flavorless and stringy.

Texture: Sticky, downy covering which some find offensive. Encloses a sea of mucous and seeds which when cooked, exudes a juice that thickens any liquid it s added to. Also gives the vegetable a slimy feel.

Purchasing: Available fresh, frozen or canned. Choose fresh that has a healthy color, tender without soft marks and bruises, no more than 4 inches long.

Storage: Fresh, extremely perishable and should be eaten as soon as purchased if not stored in paper bag in refrigerator or wrapped in a paper towel inside a perforated plastic bag in refrigerator. Will keep for 2 to 3 days or longer if frozen.

Serving Tips: Wash and scrub with vegetable brush and dry to remove stickiness. Avoid iron, or copper pans since this effects the color not taste of okra. Unless added to soup, never cut before cooking. Popular to thicken soups, stews, or ragouts. Add 10 minutes before the end of cooking process. Can also be served cold with vinaigrette or added to salad after blanching. Saut with a breadcrumb coat for 5 minutes on the stove top. Can replace asparagus and eggplant in many recipes. Goes well with tomatoes, onions, peppers, and eggplant, with spices such as curry, coriander, oregano, lemon, and vinegar.

Nutrition Facts: ½ cup

26 calories, 6 grams carbohydrates, 2 grams protein, 0 fat, and 2 grams fiber.

Vitamins/Minerals: High in vitamin C. Good source of magnesium. Also contains phosphorus, vitamin A, and folic acid.

Papaya

Name: *Papaya*

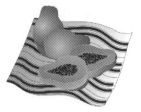

A.k.a. paw-paw, considered both a fruit and a vegetable. Spanish and Portuguese spread its culture throughout the world. Native to southern Mexico and Central America. Brazil is the leading producer in the world. Mexico is the supplier to the U.S. Crops based in Hawaii, supply to Japan and Canada.

What does it look like? Pear or cylinder shaped green skin with an orange pulp which embraces an army of black seeds that resembles peppercorn embedded in a thick, clear gelatinous film.

Taste: Sweet scented and tasting.

Texture: Like a soft melon, melt-in-the-mouth consistency.

Purchasing: Two varieties: Hawaiian and Mexican. The average papaya weighs about 1 pound. Mexican papayas can weigh up to 10 pounds.

Storage: Ripen in 3 to 5 days at room temperature. Can be stored in refrigerator up to one week. Cold temperatures halt the ripening process.

Serving Tips: Unripe papayas contain odorless whitish liquid which contains papain, an enzyme with similar properties to the bromelain in pineapples or the actidin in kiwis. Cannot be used in gelatin dishes due to the enzyme which prevents gelatinization; Left to ripen to golden-orange color and eaten fresh, chopped for salsas; pureed to use in muffin, bread and pancake mixes; as puree for smoothies, ice cream toppings, warm fruit pancake topping; decorative in salads, as garnish; often used as natural meat tenderizer; green eaten in soups and stews; goes great in yogurt or served with ham, smoked salmon. Delicious and pretty stuffed with fruit, chicken or seafood salad. The seeds can be ground and dried and used as pepper.

Nutrition Facts: ¼ medium
30 calories, 8 grams carbohydrates ½ gram protein, 0 grams fat, 2 grams fiber.

Vitamins/Minerals: High in vitamin C and potassium. Also contains vitamin A, folic acid, and magnesium. Ripe fruits contain more vitamins and minerals.

📖 CHRIS NOTES:

No reason not to eat all the time. Green papaya makes a great coleslaw old Florida favorite dish.

Passion Fruit

Name: *Passion Fruit*

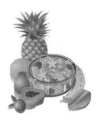

Native to Brazil, name comes from Spanish missionaries when they discovered plant in South America. They found the parts of the flowers that resembled the instruments of the Passion and the crucifixion of Christ (crown of thorns, hammers and nails.) California and Florida account for most of the domestic production in addition to South America, New Zealand, Africa, the West Indies, and Malaysia. 400 varieties, 30 edible of this fruit of the climbing vine.

What does it look like? Spherical, tear-shaped fruit, the size of an egg with a thick, smooth, lustrous inedible skin, which is yellow, orange or purple. As fruit ripens, skin becomes thinner and wrinkles. The pulp has a gelatinous texture and ranges from pinkish green to shades of orange, and yellow. It may also be white and colorless.

Taste: Combination of flavors lemon, pineapple, and guava, sweet and juicy, slightly tart, very fragrant and refreshing. Unripe fruits are very tart. Small, blackish seeds are edible.

Texture: Heavy with wrinkled skin. Gel-like interior.

Purchasing: Choose wrinkled, unbruised, and heavy fruits. Smooth skin means it s unripe.

Storage: Stored in the refrigerator, with or without skin for a week. Pulp can be frozen in an ice-cube tray and kept for several months if well wrapped.

Serving Tips: Fresh, scooped out with a spoon, sweet flavoring when added to beverages and smoothies. Also delicious in salads, yogurt, crepes, and as a topping to ice cream, and sorbets. Can also be cooked to make jams and jellies, and fermented to make alcoholic beverages.

Nutrition Facts: 4 fruits, pulp only
68 calories, 73% water, 8 grams fiber, 16 grams carbohydrates, 2 grams protein.

Vitamins/Minerals: Excellent source of vitamins C, A, and potassium. Also contains magnesium, phosphorus, folic acid, and calcium.

Health benefits: low calorie, vitamin and beta-carotene rich fruit great for weight loss, sports and overall healthy diets. Also, a very high-fiber source ideal for alleviating constipation and providing bulk to low-fiber meals such as meat, chicken, and fish. May have tranquilizing effect on the body.

CHRIS NOTES:

Once a mystery fruit, now used widely in dressings, sauces. It s even a Hawaiian Punch™ ingredient.

Persimmon

Name: *Persimmon*

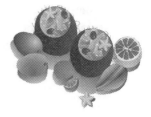

Cultivated in China for centuries, sometimes called the apple of the Orient. In Japan, it is the national fruit called kaki. Introduced to California in the 1870s. Hundreds of varieties classified into two main groups—the Asian hachiya and fuyu and the American which grows wild in the southeastern United States.

What does it look like? 1-inch to 3-inch, spherical or acorn-like, smooth skin, light-yellow orange to brilliant orange red fruit, with up to 8 large, brown inedible seeds. Like a tomato.

Taste: Unripe, the hachiya is astringent and inedible. Must be consumed ripe when it turns from green to bright red.

Texture: Like more firm, mealy tomato like texture.

Purchasing: Avoid green or yellow fruit.

Storage: Will ripen at room temperature. To hasten process place in paper bag either alone or with another fruit which produces ethylene gas such as an apple or banana. Keep ripe persimmons in the refrigerator. May be frozen whole or pureed. Add 1½ tbsp. of lemon juice to 1-cup of puree to prevent discoloration.

Serving Tips: Delicious raw, but only when very ripe. Added to cakes, cookies, brownies, and breads. Puree can be used as sauce for poultry, or desserts. Great for rice, couscous, seafood, and poultry dishes. Can be canned or dried.

Nutrition Facts: ½ fruit
59 calories, 16 grams carbohydrate, 0 grams protein, 0 grams fat, 3 grams fiber.

Vitamins/Minerals: Great source of vitamin A and potassium. Also contains vitamin C.

📖 CHRIS NOTES:

There are two types of persimmons, astringent and non-astringent. For less astringent taste, eat very overripe.

Pineapple

Name: *Pineapple*

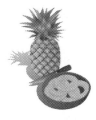

Called pina, because of its likeness to pine cone. Resemblance inspired the English word pineapple. Cultivated in South America and West Indies since ancient times. Christopher Columbus discovered during his voyage to Guadeloupe in 1493 and brought it to Europe where it spread to many parts of the world on ships that carried it as a protection against scurvy. The Portuguese and Spanish introduced it to their Asian colonies. Main producers today are Thailand and Philippines.

Taste: Sweet, but unlike other fruits does not become sweeter after harvest.

Texture: Fibrous and juicy.

Purchasing: Cayenne, Queen, Red Spanish and Pernambuco varieties. Buy heavy for size, pleasantly aromatic, with fresh, deep green leaves, and yields to slight pressure of fingers. Strong odor means fruit has begun to ferment. Cayenne variety used for canning. Red Spanish is suited to shipping.

Storage: Refrigerated in plastic bag after purchase. Cut may be kept sealed in refrigerator 1 week.

Serving Tips: Fresh in salads. Include in muffins, cakes, and breads. Canned, use in marinades for tenderizing meats and poultry. Not used in gelatins, yogurt, and cottage cheese because its digestive enzyme bromelain breaks down the protein in these foods and makes them watery. However, canned or boiled varieties can be used since the enzyme is degraded by heat.

Nutrition Facts: ½ cup
30 calories, 10 grams carbohydrates, 0 protein, 0 fat, 1 g fiber.

Vitamins/Minerals: vitamin C, potassium, folate, and magnesium.

Plantain

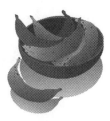

Name: *Plantain*

Fruit of the banana tree, referred to as cooking banana. Native to Malaysia, a staple in many regions. Common in India, West Indies, and South America.

Taste: Cooked as a fruit then bland to sweet as sweet potato. Will take on flavor of seasonings of dish.

Texture: 10 to 15 inches long, green skin thicker than banana, like a banana, firmer.

Purchasing: Firm and intact, brownish and black on skin acceptable does not affect taste.

Storage: Keep at room temperature, refrigerate only when very ripe.

Serving Tips: used as a side dish, cooked in soups or stews, fried, saut ed, boiled.

Nutrition Facts: 3½ oz.
122 calories, 32 grams carb, 1 gram protein, less than 1 gram fat, 2 grams fiber.

Vitamins/Minerals: potassium, good of vitamins C, B6, and magnesium. Also vitamins A and folic acid.

Pomegranate

Name: *Pomegranate*

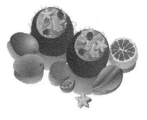

Fruit with a colorful history, name derived from Old French term pome for apple and grenate for many—seeded. Native to Europe and Asia. Long celebrated in art and literature. Seeds are the Hebrew sign of fertility. The fruit was once part of the decoration on King Solomon's temple pillars. Brought to the new world by Spanish missionaries in 16th century.

Taste: Three varieties one sour, two that are sweet.

Texture: Round fruit, the size of large orange with protruding crown and smooth leathery, yellowish-pink to red skin. Contains hundreds of ruby colored seeds that are individually encased in a translucent red juicy pulp. Each seed is sweet to tart, separated by creamy, colored compartments that are bitter. Seeds and pulp are edible.

Purchasing: Available in United States from October to December. Buy heavy-for-size fruits, with slightly soft crown and shiny skin.

Storage: Refrigerate up to 2 months. Store in a cool, dark place for a month.

Serving Tips: Labor-intensive to eat. After peeling skin, seeds can be removed individually, or the fruit can be cut in half and the seeds scooped away with a spoon. Seeds are used for garnish, in salads, or drinks. Dried it can be used as substitute for raisins in cakes. Grenadine, light syrup used in adult and kid s cocktail called Shirley Temples are a 7-Up and grenadine mixture. Pomegranate molasses is used in Mediterranean and Middle Eastern cooking.

Nutrition Facts: 1 fruit
105 calories, 26 grams carbohydrates, 1 gram protein, 0 grams fat, 1 gram fiber.

Vitamins/Minerals: Potassium, B6, and vitamin C.

Prickly Pear

Name: *Prickly Pear*

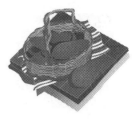

Originated in Mexico and Caribbean, as many as 1,000 species, from the cactus family. Ripe fruits collected by American Indians. Older pads used for livestock feed. Spanish explorers introduced plants to Spain. National fruit of Israel called Sharon's fruit.

Taste: Mildly sweet, juicy and fragrant with tiny small crunchy seeds.

Texture: Yellow to dark-red flesh is juicy.

Purchasing: Bright, firm fruit. Be careful to watch for prickly spine.

Storage: Left at room temperature to ripen. When ripe, fruits yield when gently pressed

Serving Tips: Fresh with a sprinkle of key lime, diced, and used as topping for frozen desserts, and pancakes. Puree can be added to muffin mixes, smoothies, and coulis.

Nutrition Facts: 1 fruit
44 calories, 10 grams carbohydrates, 1 gram protein and fat, 4 grams fiber.

Vitamins/Minerals: vitamin C, potassium, calcium, and magnesium.

CHRIS NOTES:
In Mexico, fruits grown on plant with round pads which are also commonly consumed after careful removal of cactus needles.

Quince

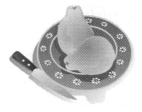

Name: *Quince*

"Native to Iran, popular among Greeks and Romans. The Greeks believed it warded off bad luck and valued it as sign of love and fertility. Used in wedding rites. Romans used its' essential oil in perfumes.

Taste: Raw it is bitter because of high tannin content. Bitterness disappears with cooking however, serve immediately because it oxidizes quickly. You can also sprinkle the fruit with a vitamin C-rich juice like lemon or lime juice to prevent bad aftertaste.

Texture: Like apple or pear.

Purchasing: Buy plump, firm and undamaged, partially yellow skin. Avoid hard, green fruits.

Storage: Ripen in cold, 57 to 67... F temperatures. Store at room temperature, wrapped individually and refrigerated. Freezes well after cooked

Serving Tips: Used in jams, jellies, (due to the large amount of pectin which is a thickening agent). Eat like baked apple, use in stuffing or in baked goods for texture, or for vitamin C and potassium enrichment. Serve with meat and poultry or as fruit compote.

Nutrition Facts: about ½ cup (3½ oz.)
57 calories, 15 grams carbohydrates, less than 1 gram protein and 1 gram fat, 1.7 gram fiber.

Vitamins/Minerals: Potassium, vitamin C, and copper.

⦿ *Nutrition Nugget*
Believed to be good for GI system. Quince can take the place of apples in your favorite jelly recipe.

Sapodilla

Name: *Sapodilla*

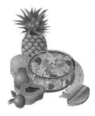

Originated in Yucatan peninsula of Mexico, northern Belize. Prized by the Aztecs who called the fruit "tzapotl" from which the Spanish renamed it sapodilla. Main producers are Central American countries, India, Indonesia, California, and Florida.

Taste: Sweet like honey, and apricots when ripe. Astringent and unpalatable when unripe.

Texture: Melt in the mouth texture with 3 to 12 hard shiny black seeds. Ingestion of more than six seeds can cause abdominal pain and vomiting.

Purchasing: Fresh, the tree bears fruit in May through September. Buy firm, heavy for size, with no blemishes.

Storage: Unripe should be left to ripen at room temperature and refrigerated after ripening.

Serving Tips: The ideal dessert fruit. Used for salads, raw snack, in desserts such as ice cream and sorbet, and dried in India.

Nutrition Facts: 1 fruit
141 calories, 34 grams carbohydrates, 1 gram protein, 2 grams fat, 9 grams fiber.

Vitamins/Minerals: Calcium, potassium, vitamins A, C and folic acid.

📖 CHRIS NOTES:
Intensely sweet fruit, can be cooked or used fresh as a topping on ice cream. Sap from tree was originally used for chewing gum until 1960s when synthetic gum products were developed.

Tomatillo

Name: *Tomatillo*

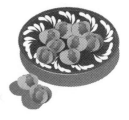

Small green tomato, little tomato in Spanish. Native of Mexico, grows wild in California. Can be grown as far north as central Midwestern U.S. Belongs to nightshade family, and is actually a fruit.

Taste: Tangy, lemony flavor.

Texture: Firmer than tomato, flesh is pale-green or yellow, depending on degree of ripeness.

Purchasing: Firm fruits that just fill the husks are best. Remove husk before consuming. Canned also available.

Storage: In the refrigerator, unwashed or in a plastic or paper bag, for 3 weeks or longer.

Serving Tips: Cooking enhances the flavor even though it is often eaten raw in salads and salsas.

Nutrition Facts: ½ c. chopped
21 calories, 4 grams carbohydrates 1 gram protein, 1 gram fat, 1 gram fiber.

Vitamins/Minerals: Potassium and vitamin C.

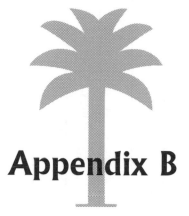

Appendix B

Tropical Diet: Food Groups and Servings©

Detox Phase 1

Food Group	Pro (Gms)	Carb (Gms)	Fat (Gms)	Energy (Calorie) Levels*			
				1000	1200	1500	1800
Milk or Milk Substitutes 100 calories/serving	8	12	varies 1	0 based	0 based	0	0
Fruit 60 calories/serving		15		5	6	7	8
Vegetables 50 calories/cup	4	10	varies	3c+	3c+	3c+	4c+
Grains/Starches 80 calories/serving	3	15	varies	2	3	4	5
Protein/ Meat Substitutes 55 cal/serving	7-10		varies	6	8	10	12
Fat 45 calories/serving			5	3	3	4	5
Total Calories*:				987	1202	1462	1778
Grams (g)/Percent % calories from:							
Carbohydrates				135g/55%	165g/55%	195g/53%	235g/53%
Protein				60g/24%	77g/26%	94g/26%	115g/26%
Fat				23g/21%	26g/19%	34g/21%	42g/21%

*Approximate calories based on The American Diabetic/Dietetic Association exchanges using the Compu-Cal/Pro Nutrition Assessment Computer. Always check Tropical Diet™ Food Lists for portion size.

Lean Plan: high protein, low, simple-carbohydrate, moderate fat

Food Group	Pro (Gms)	Carb (Gms)	Fat (Gms)	Energy (Calorie) Levels*				
				1000	1200	1500	1800	2000
Milk or Milk Substitutes 100 calories/serving	8	12	varies 1	1	2	2	3	3
Fruit 60 calories/serving		15		4 based	5 based	6	6	7
Vegetables 50 calories/cup	4	10	varies	2c	3c	3c	3c	3c
Grains/Starches 80 calories/serving	3	15	varies	2	2	3	4	4
Protein/ Meat Substitutes 55 cal/serving	7-10		varies	8	10	12	13	15
Fat 45 calories/serving			5	3	3	3	4	6
Total Calories*:				1025	1295	1510	1753	1977
Grams (g)/Percent % calories from:								
Carbohydrates				122g/48%	159g/49%	189g/50%	216g/49%	231g/47%
Protein				78g/30%	104g/32%	121g/32%	139g/32%	153g/31%
Fat				25g /22%	27g/19%	30g/18%	37g/19%	49g/22%

*Approximate calories based on The American Diabetic/Dietetic Association exchanges using the Compu-Cal/Pro Nutrition Assessment Computer. Always check Tropical Diet™ Food Lists for portion size.

*A*thlete Plan: high-carbohydrate, moderate protein, low fat

Food Group	Pro (Gms)	Carb (Gms)	Fat (Gms)	Energy (Calorie) Levels*				
				1200	1500	1800	2000	2400
Milk or Milk Substitutes 100 calories/serving	8	12	varies 1	2 based	3 based	3	3	3
Fruit 60 calories/serving		15		6	7	8	8	8
Vegetables 50 calories/cup	4	10	varies	3c	3c	3c	3c	3c
Grains/Starches 80 calories/serving	3	15	varies	3	4	5	6	9
Protein/ Meat Substitutes 55 cal/serving	7-10		varies	5	6	8	10	12
Fat 45 calories/serving			5	2	3	4	4	6
Total Calories*:				1206	1449	1769	1969	2331
Grams (g)/Percent% calories from:								
Carbohydrates				189g/63%	216g/60%	261g/509%	276g/56%	321g/55%
Protein				72g/24%	90g/25%	107g/24%	124g/25%	147g/25%
Fat				18g/13%	25g/15%	33g/17%	41g/19%	51g/20%

*Approximate calories based on The American Diabetic/Dietetic Association exchanges using the Compu-Cal/Pro Nutrition Assessment Computer. Always check Tropical Diet™ Food Lists for portion size.

Basic Plan: protein, fat and carbohydrate balance

Food Group	Pro (Gms)	Carb (Gms)	Fat (Gms)	Energy (Calorie) Levels*			
				1200	1500	1800	2000
Milk or Milk Substitutes 100 calories/serving	8	12	varies	2	2	2	3
Fruit 60 calories/serving		15		4 based	5 based	6	6
Vegetables 50 calories/cup	4	10	varies	2c	2c	2c	3c
Grains/Starches 80 calories/serving	3	15	varies	2	3	4	4
Protein/ Meat Substitutes 55 cal/serving	7-10		varies	8	10	12	14
Fat 45 calories/serving			5	5	6	8	8
Total Calories*:				1195	1455	1760	1914
Grams (g)/Percent% calories from:							
Carbohydrates				134g/45%	164g/45%	194g/44%	206g/43%
Protein				86g/29%	103g/28%	120g/27%	142g/30%
Fat				35g/26%	43g/27%	56g/29%	58g/27%

*Approximate calories based on The American Diabetic/Dietetic Association exchanges using the Compu-Cal/Pro Nutrition Assessment Computer. Always check Tropical Diet™ Food Lists for portion size.

Appendix C

Recommended Resources

BOOKS

Berning, Jacqueline R. and Steen, Suzanne Nelson. *Nutrition For Sport and Exercise,* 2nd edition. Aspen Publishers, Maryland, 1998. *For serious athletes, athletic or personal trainers, coaches, and nutritionists, an advanced-level, comprehensive guide to sports nutrition.*

Burke, V. *Caribbean Kitchen.* Simon & Schuster, London, 2000. *Colorful and authentic book by Jamaican and Director of Walkerswood Company, a Caribbean based foods and Spice Company (see websites) and Chef Euten Lindsay.*

Canadian Dietetic Association, *Healthy Pleasures.* Macmillan, Canada. 1995. *A compilation of delicious, and easy-to-prepare healthy recipes from Canada's nutrition experts, registered dietitians and executive chefs.*

Clark, Nancy. *Sports Nutrition Guidebook,* Third Edition. Human Kinetics, Illinois, 2003. *A best-selling nutritionist shares her third edition of her informative sports nutrition book.*

Dewitt, D. Wilan, MJ. *Callaloo, Calypso and Carnival, the Cuisines of Trinidad and Tobago.* 1993. The Crossing Press, Freedom, California, 1993. *A fun cookbook with insight into the foods, preparation and islands of this great cuisine. Includes glossary, mail order resources and tourism information.*

Dorfman, Lisa. *The Vegetarian Sports Nutrition Guide.* John Wiley & Sons, New York, 2000. *A must have, the only book to address the essential nutritional needs of athletes which highlights vegetarian sports nutrition. Features 17 Olympian, world class and elite athletes in football, wrestling, swimming, basketball, skating, triathlon, running, equestrian and curling. Recipes, diets and supplement information included.*

Duyff, Roberta Larson. *American Dietetic Association Complete Food and Nutrition Guide, 2nd Edition.* John Wiley & Sons, 2002. *An invaluable and comprehensive must-have diet and nutrition resource from nutrition expert and registered dietitian.*

Janzan, K. *The ABC of the Creative Caribbean Cookery.* Macmillan-Caribbean. 1994. *A former charter chef shares her insight on many of the Caribbean islands, their customs and traditional dishes.*

Litt, Ann Selkowitz. *The College Student's Guide to Eating Well on Campus.* Tulip Hill Press. *This 256-page book is chock full of information for students and grown ups alike. Available through Amazon.com.*

MacLauchlan, Andrew, and Flynn, Donna K. *Tropical Deserts. Recipes for Exotic Fruits, Nuts, and Spices.* Macmillan, New York. 1997. *The most incredible tropical dessert recipes and photos demonstrate the gourmet side of tropical cuisine from the well-versed pastry chef.*

Milton, Jane. *Mexican Healthy ways with a Favorite Cuisine.* Annes Publishing Limited. 2003. *A colorful and comprehensive guide to the foods, traditional dishes and preparation methods of Mexico.*

Pitkin, Julia M. *Great Chefs of the Caribbean.* Cumberland House Publishing. Nashville, Tennessee, 2000. *146 recipes from more than 44 chefs from Mexico and 17 islands, an advanced cookbook with incredible recipes and photos.*

Ponichtera BJ. *Quick and Healthy Recipes and Ideas.* Volume I. 1991 and Quick and Healthy Recipes and Ideas. Volume II. 1995. *Two of my favorite easy-to-prepare, healthy cookbooks ideal for singles and families written by a nutrition expert and registered dietitian. Over 250,000 copies in print. Winner of the Benjamin Franklin Award.* 503-296-1875 or ScaleDown Publishing 1519 Hermits Way, The Dalles, Oregon 97058.

Rahamut, W. *Caribbean Flavors.* Macmillan Publishers, Caribbean. 2002. *A beautiful woman, TV personality, and food consultant from Trinidad shares an authentic and easy- to-follow cookbook.*

Rare Fruit Council, International Inc., Miami, Florida. *Rare and Exotic Tropical Fruit Recipes.* 1981. *Old but classic, and still available from The Fruit and Spice Park in Homestead, Florida is a handy and informative guide and recipe book for tropical fruits.*

Robinson, Jan. *Slim to Shore Cookbook.* Ship to Shore, Inc. US Virgin Islands. *This yacht captain and cooking diva is the author of this fabulous healthy Caribbean style cookbook and five other best-selling cookbooks. You won't find these books in the bookstores. Call 1-800-338-6072.*

Shields, Donna. *Caribbean Light.* Doubleday, New York, 1998. *A delicious and comprehensive nutritional, culinary and humorous look at Caribbean cuisine with an enormous amount of personal insight shared by this registered dietitian/culinary expert. Island cuisine without the excesses of fat and sugars seasoned just right!*

Van Aken, Norman. *The Great Exotic Fruit Book.* Ten Speed Press, Berkeley, California, 1995. *One of the world's greatest chefs and pioneer in New World Cuisine, this book describes and shows some of the most delicious tropical fruits and recipes also available at his restaurants and featured in his cookbooks, posters and postcards. You need to try his cuisine just once to understand his gift and appreciation for these tropical foods and spices. Call 800-841-book.*

Walsh R. and McCarthy J. *Traveling Jamaica with Knife, Fork, and Spoon, A Righteous Guide to Jamaican Cookery.* Freedom, California, 1995. *Authentic narrated, and easy-to-prepare recipes from this Jamaican Executive Chef.*

Whittaker, Anne-Marie. *Treasures of my Caribbean Kitchen.* Macmillan Publishers, 1999. *This Barbados based author shares her recipes and island insight in a delicious cookbook. Native Treasures hot sauces and products are also available through her website www.native-treasures.com.*

Woodruff S. *Secrets of Cooking for Long Life.* Avery Publishing Group, New York, 1999. *Best-selling cookbook author and registered dietitian shares basic nutrition and an army of recipes with the nutritional analysis provided for helping you prepare and stick to any diet program. Photos included.*

Nutrition, Food, and Fitness Newsletters and Organizations

American Dietetic Association.
The largest group of nutrition experts, approximately 70,000 educators, chefs, clinicians, consultants, counselors, foodservice executives, sports nutritionists, researchers, and private practitioners. Website offers cutting-edge dietary info and referral service. 1-800-877-1600 or website: *www.eatright.org.*

Nutrition Action Healthletter.
Published 10 times a year by the *Center for Science in the Public Interest. A*

must-have, cutting-edge, consumer friendly newsletter on health and nutrition issues often highlighted in popular press. Contact circ@cspinet.org or FAX 202-265-4954.

Environmental Nutrition Newsletter
Monthly newsletter featuring at least 15 cutting-edge reports food safety, research updates, expert opinions, and sensible, practical guidance from registered dietitians (R.D.). Call 800-829-5384 or *enu@palmcoastd.com.*

Food & Fitness Advisor
Weill Medical College of Cornell University monthly newsletter provides timely news and medical information. Call: 800-829-2505 or email: *Foodandfit@ palmcoastd.com.*

Nutrition Action Health Letter
Center For Science In the Public Interest. Published 10 times a year by a nonprofit health-advocacy group. A practical and cutting-edge newsletter on all health, food, and nutrition topics. *www.cspinet.com.*

Supermarket Savvy Newsletter
A comprehensive newsletter and website which provides nutrition information, trends and product information. A must have for the food savvy tropical dieter. *SupermarketSavvy.com.*

Tufts University Health & Nutrition Letter
A monthly food, fitness, and health newsletter which provides the latest research, and expert opinion on nutrition, health, disease, and food-related issues. Call: 800-274-7581 Outside U.S. 386-447-6336 Website: *www.healthletter.tufts.edu.*

Websites and Companies for Ordering or Locating Tropical Foods

Canned Food Alliance. *www.Mealtime.org.*
With more than 1500 canned food items, this website offers expert nutrition advice, recipes, dietary information and research.

Fairchild Gardens, Miami, Florida. Tropical Fruit Pavilion.
The first in the U.S. offers botanical and tropical research, tours, programs, and memberships. www.fairchildgarden.org.

Fruit and Spice Park. *Botanical tours, workshops, spa days, seminars, and events— Redland Natural Arts Festival, Farm and Garden Show and Thai-Asian Festival. Specialty store.* 305-247-5727 *fsp@miamidade.gov.*

Frieda s Exotic and Healthy Foods. Los Angeles, California.
Frieda's®, Inc., is the nation's leading marketer and distributor of specialty produce. The company supplies grocery retailers, wholesalers, and food service distributors with more than 500 different items through its branded product lines: Frieda's®, Cocina de Frieda®, Asian Specialties™, and Vegetarian

Solutions™ for meatless meal ideas for the produce. Website has over 500 items, recipe club, store, and retailer information. In addition, the company has a mail-order division, Frieda's By Mail that serves the foodservice industry, special orders and gift baskets. 4465 Corporate Center Dr., Los Alamitos, CA 90720, 714-826-6100 or toll-free call: 800-241-1771 Website: *www.friedas.com.*

J.R. Brooks, & Son, Tropical Food Companies, and Farms Inc. Homestead, Florida. P.O. Box 900160, Homestead, Florida 33090 800-327-4833.

Ocho Rios™ snacks and foods from Jamaica. Distributed by: Ocho Rios Miami, Inc. 305-326-1734. *www.ochoriosja.com.*

Melissa s World Variety Produce. *Offers a variety of organic and exotic fruits and vegetables, gourmet food, corporate gift baskets, and holiday treats online and delivered to your door. Products also available at health food and specialty/gourmet markets. Website is chock-full-of incredible and delicious food, cultural, and cooking information.* 800-588-0151. Website: *www.melissas.com.*

Robert is Here Fruit Stand. *Exotic and tropical fruits, vegetables, dressings, sauces, mustards, chutneys, pickles, preserves, jams, syrups, and honey.* 305-246-1592 or *www.robertishere.com.*

Tropical Fruit and Vegetable Society of the Redlands, Inc. Homestead, Florida. *Membership/monthly meetings.* 24801 SW 187 Avenue, Homestead, Florida 33031

Tropical Fruit Growers of South Florida, Homestead, Fl. *The history, availability, handling and identification of tropical fruits. www.fl-ag.com/tropical/*

University of Florida, Institute of Food and Agricultural Services (IFAS) *Tropical Research and Education Center, Homestead, Florida. Seminars, books, academic programs.* 18905 SW 280 Street, Homestead, Florida 330131 305-246-7001 *www.trec.ifas.ufl.edu.*

Taste of the Tropics from Down Under. Comprehensive website from Austrialia offering information on exotic fruit, seafood, nutrition, recipes, regional cuisines, and local markets. www.tropicalfruitworld.com www.australian tropicalfoods.com.

Walkerswood Marketing and Products-North America. *Spices, sauce, and canned Caribbean foods.* Website: *www.walkerswood.com* Email: *wwoodna@bellsouth.net.*

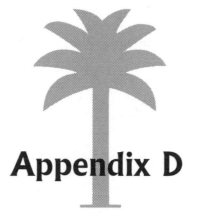

Appendix D

References

Acheson KJ, Gremaud G, Meirim I, Montigon F, Krebs Y, Fay LS, Gay LJ, Schneiter P, Schindler C, Tappy L. Metabolic effects of caffeine in humans: lipid oxidation or futile cycling? *American Journal of Clinical Nutrition,* 2004; 79(1): 40—6.

Adom KK, Liu RH. Antioxidant activity of grains. *Journal of Agricultural Food Chemistry* 2002; 50 (21): 6182—7.

Alford BB, Blankenship AC, Hagen RD. The effects of variations in carbohydrates, protein, and fat content of the diet upon weight loss, blood values, and nutrient intake of adult obese women. *Journal of American Dietetic Association* 1990; 90(4): 534—40.

Shaw, P., Chan, H., and Nagy, S. *All about Citrus and Subtropical Fruits.* Ortho Books. 1985.

Anne-Marie Whittaker. *Treasures of my Caribbean Kitchen.* Macmillan Publishers, 1999.

Andrew MacLauchlan and Donna K. Flynn. *Tropical Desserts .Recipes for Exotic Fruits, Nuts, and Spices.* A Simon and Schuster Macmillan Company New York, NY 1997.

Antinoro L., Food and herbs to keep blood moving, prevent circulatory problems. *Environmental Nutrition* 2000, Feb 3.

Astrup A., Dietary approaches to reducing body weight. Baillieres Best Practical *Research in Clinical Endocrinology Metabolism.* 1999; 13(1): 109—120.

Astrup A, Astrup A, Buemann B, Flint A, Raben A. Low-fat diets and energy balance: how does the evidence stand in 2002 *Proctors of Nutrition Society* 2002; 61(2): 299—309.

Bazzano LA, He J, Ogden LG, Loria C, Vupputuri S, Myers L, Whelton PK. Legume consumption and risk of coronary heart disease in US men and women: NHANES I Epidemiologic Follow-up Study. *Archive of Internal Medicine* 2001; 161(21): 2573—78.

Bazzano LA, He J, Ogden LG, Loria C, Vupputuri S, Myers L, Whelton PK. Legume consumption and risk of coronary heart disease in US men and women: NHANES I Epidemiologic Follow-up Study. *American Journal of Nutrition* 2002; 76 (1): 93—9.

Bernstein M. Hot cocoa tops red wine and tea in antioxidants; may be healthier choice. *www.eurekalert.org/pub*, 2003.

Betty s body shaping *www.betty@seidosydney.com.au* and 2003; 2 (2): 1—4.

Bryant J., Fat is a $34 billion business at *www.bizjournals.com/atlanta/stories/2001/09/24/story4.html,* 2003.

Bourne, MJ, Lennox GW, Seddon SA. *Fruits and Vegetables of the Caribbean.* Macmillan Education Limited, 1988.

Burke, V. *Caribbean Kitchen.* Simon & Schuster, London, 2000.

Canadian Dietetic Association, *Healthy Pleasures.* Macmillan Canada Toronto 1995.

Canned Food Alliance. *Whoever Said Fresh is Best May Have To Eat Those Words* brochure, 2004.

Choo JJ. Green tea reduces body fat accretion caused by high-fat diet in rats through beta-adrenoceptor activation of thermogenisis in brown adipose tissue. *Journal of Nutritional Biochemistry* 2003; 14(11): 671—6.

Chu YF, Sun J, Wu X, Liu RH. Antioxidant and antiproliferative activities of common vegetables. *Journal of Agricultural Food Chemistry* 2002; 50(23): 6910—16.

Cooper A, Poirier S, Murphy M, Oswald MJ, Procise C, Bobroff LB, Bobroff S. South Florida Tropicals: Black Sapote. http:// edis.ifas.ufl.edu/Body HE609.

Cox BD,. Seasonal Consumption of Salad Vegetables and Fresh Fruit in relation to the Development of Cardiovascular Disease and Cancer. *Public Health Nutrition,* 2000.

Crovetti R, Porrini M, Santangelo A, Testolin G. The influence of thermic effect of food on satiety. *European Journal of Clinical Nutrition* 1998; 52(7): 482—488.

Dewitt, D. Wilan MJ. *Callaloo, Calypso and Carnival, the Cuisines of Trinidad and Tobago.* The Crossing Press, Freedom, California, 1993.

DeAngelis T, Family size portions for one, *www.apa.org/monitor/jan04/family.html,* 2003.

Dole Food Company. *Encyclopedia of Foods, A Guide to Healthy Nutrition.* Academic Press San Diego, California, 2002.

Dorfman, Lisa. *The Vegetarian Sports Nutrition Guide.* John Wiley & Sons, New York, 2000.

Driskell, J, and Wolinsky, Ira. *Nutritional Assessment of Athletes.* CRC Press, Boca Raton. 2002 pp213—222.

Dulloo AG, Duret C, Rohrer D, Girardier L, Mensi N, Fathi M, Chantre VJ. Efficacy of a green tea extracts rich in polyphenols and caffeine in increasing 24—h energy expenditure and fat oxidation in humans. *American Journal of Clinical Nutrition* 1999; 70 (6): 1040—5

Ed Landry. Caribbean Adventures. *Classic Cajun Cooking and Tales from the Reign of the Pirates.* Adlai House Publishing Lakeside, CA, 1994.

Ellsworth JL, Kushi LH, Folsom AR, Frequent nut intake and risk of death from coronary heart disease and all causes in postmenopausal women: the Iowa Women s Health Study. *JAMA.* 2003; 290(1): 38—39.

Fabicant, F. Tropical Paradise on a Plate: Chef s Promote Taste of Exotic Fruits. *Nation's Restaurant News,* 1998.

Farnsworth E, Luscombe ND, Noakes M, Wittert G, Argyiou E, Clifton PM. Effect of a high-protein, energy-restricted diet on body composition, Glycemic control, and lipid concentrations in overweight and obese hyperinsulinemic men and women. *American Journal of Clinical Nutrition* 2000; 78: 31—39.

Finer N. Low-Calorie diets and sustained weight loss. Obesity Research 2001; 9(4): 290S—294S.

Florida Department of Agriculture and Consumer Services. *Tropical Fruit Cookbook* Tallahassee, Florida.

Florida Lime Administrative Committee. Limes, Limes, Limes . . . Florida s Juicy Fruit Brochure.

Food Insight Fad diets: Look Before You Leap *www.ificinfo.health.org.*

Ford Es, Mokdad AH. Fruit and vegetable consumption and diabetes mellitus incidence among US adults. *Preventive Medicine* 2001; 32(1): 33—39.

Fortin, F. *The Visual Food Encyclopedia.* Macmillan, USA, 1996.

Foster-Powell K, Holt SHA, Brand-Miller JC.International table of Glycemic index and Glycemic index load values. *American Journal of Clinical Nutrition* 2002; 76: 5—56.

Friedrick, J. When it comes to Tropical Flavors, fruit has the Appeal. *Gourmet News,* 2003.

Friedrick, J. Could Dragonfruit fuel a new Product Firestorm? *Gourmet News,* 2003.

Fujiki H, Suganuma M, Okabe S, Sueoka E, Suga K, Imai K, Nakachi K, Kimura S. Mechanistic findings of green tea as cancer preventive for humans. *Proctor of Society of Experimental Biological Medicine* 1999; 220(4): 225—8.

Grobbee DE, Rinm EB, Giobannucci E, Coiditz G, Stampfer M, Willett W. Coffee, Caffeine and cardiovascular disease in man. *New England Journal of Medicine* 1990; 323 (15): 1026—32.

Hart K, Greenwood H, Truby H. Pound for pound? Comparing the costs incurred by subjects following four commercially available weight loss programs. *Journal of Human Nutrition and Dietetics* 2003; 16(5): 365.

Hasler CM, Kundrat S, Wool D, Functional foods and cardiovascular disease. *Current Atherosclerosis* Rep. 2000; 2(6): 467—75.

Hays NP, Starling RD, Xiaolan L, Sullivan DH, Trappe TA, Fluckey JD, Evans WJ, Effects of an Ad libitum low fat, high-carbohydrate diet on body weight, body composition, and fat distribution in older men and women. *Archives of Internal Medicine* 2004; 164: 210—217.

Herber D, Bownerman S. *What Color is Your Diet?* Regan Books, Harper Collins Publisher, 2001.

Henry and Emery. Spiced foods and metabolic rate. *Human Nutrition: Clinical Nutrition* 1986; 40C: 165—68.

High Protein Diet and Diabetes Mellitus. *American Journal of Clinical Nutrition* 2003; 78(4):734—41.

Hope S, Warshaw M.MSc., R.D. Craving Chinese? Italian? How to eat healthfully when dining out. *Environmental Nutrition* 2001 May 6.

Holt SH, Belargy HJ, Lawton CL, Blundell JE. The effects of high-carbohydrates vs. high-fat breakfast on feelings of fullness and alertness, and subsequent food intake. *International Journal of Food Science and Nutrition* 1999; 50(1): 13—28.

Hutton, W. *Tropical Vegetables.* Periplus Nature Guides. 1996.

Jane Milton. *Mexican Healthy ways with a Favorite Cuisine.* Annes Publishing Limited, 2003.

Janzan K. *The ABC of the Creative Caribbean Cookery.* Macmillan Press 1994.

Jeanne Ambrose. The Quince essential. *Better Homes and Gardens* 2003 Dec 230.

Jequier E, Bray GA. Low fat diets are preferred. *American Journal of Medicine* 2002; 113(9B): 41S—46S.

Jiang R, Manson JE, Stampfer MJ, Liu S, Willett WC, Hu FB. Nut and peanut butter consumption and risk of type 2 diabetes in women. *Preventive Medicine* 1999; 28(4): 333—9.

Joffe M, Robertson A. The potential contribution of increased vegetable and fruit consumption to health gain in the European Union. *Public Health Nutrition* 2001; 4(4): 893—901.

Johnson CS, Day CS, Swan PD. Postprandial thermo genesis is increased 100% on a high protein low fat diet versus a high carbohydrate, low fat diet in healthy, young women. American Journal of Collective Nutrition and *www.jacn.org.*

Johnstone AM, Stubbs RJ, Harbron CG. Effect of overfeeding macronutrients on day to day food intake in man. *European Journal of Clinical Nutrition* 1996; 50(7): 418—430.

JR Brooks & Son. *Teaching with Tropicals,* brochure, 1986.

JR Brooks & Son, Tropical Food Companies and Farms Inc. Homestead, Florida.

Julia M. Pitkin. *Great Chefs of the Caribbean.* Cumberland House Publishing. Division of GCI, Inc. 2000.

Karetnick, J. *In Good Taste, the Spices of Island Life.* Air Jamaica Escapades. 2002.

Kenney JJ. 10 Best Reasons a Low-Carb Diet is Wrong. Excerpted from the January 2000 issue of communicating food for health and the low-carb fad diet 2000. *www.foodandhealth.com.*

Kiwi Fruit: Vibrant Green and Gold Kiwifruit Boast Key Nutrients. Environmental Nutrition 2003; 26: 8 and *www.environmentalnutrition.com.*

Komatsu T, Nakamori M, Kamatsu K, Hosoda K, Okamura M, Toyama K, Tehikura Y, Sakai T, Kunii D, Yamamoto S. Oolong tea increases energy metabolism in Japanese females. *Journal of Medical Investigation* 2003; 50 (3—4): 170—5.

La Vecchia C, Tavani A. Fruit and Vegetables, and human cancer. *European Journal of Cancer Prevention* 1998; 7(1): 3—8.

Lavedrine F, Zmirou D, Ravel A, Balducci F, Alary J. Blood Cholesterol and walnut consumption: a cross-sectional survey in France. *Preventive Medicine* 1999; 28(4): 333—9.

Leitzmann MF, Willett WC, Rimm EB, Stampfer MJ, Spiegelman D, Coidit GA, Giovannucci E. A perspective study of coffee consumption and the risk of symptomatic gallstone disease in men. *JAMA* 1999; 281(22): 2106—12.

Lepke J. Pump up potassium to keep blood pressure low, prevent stroke. *Environmental Nutrition* 1999; 22: 2.

Liebman, B. Hurley J. Pickers can be choosers. *Nutrition Action Healthletter,* 2003; June: 13—14.

Liu S, Manson JE, Lee IM, Cole SR, Hennkens CH, Willett WC, Buring JE. Fruit and vegetable intake and risk of cardiovascular disease: the women s health study. *American Journal of Clinical Nutrition* 2000; 72(4): 922—8.

Lorenza De Medici. *A Passion for Fruit.* Pavilion Books, Limited London, 1999.

Maron DJ, Lu GP, Cai NS, Wu ZG, Li YH, Chen H, Zhu JQ, Jin XJ, Woute BC, Zhao J. Cholesterol lowering effect of a theaflavin-enriched green tea extract: a randomized controlled trial. *Archives of Internal Medicine* 2003; 163 (12): 1448—53.

McArdle WD, Katch FI, Katch VL. *Sports and Exercise Nutrition.* Lippincott Williams and Wilkins, 1999.

MacLauchlan. Tropical Desserts. Macmillan, New York. 1997.

Mahan K. and Escott-Stump S. *Food, Nutrition, and Diet Therapy.* Elsevier, Pennsylvania, 2004.

Meltzer W. The Fruit Bowl. *Nutrition Action Healthletter* at *www.cspinet.org/nah/ fantfruit/htm.*

Miami Herald: Plan for America s new diet: less sprawl, less fat, less frenzy at *www.miami.com/mld/miamiherald/news/5959760.html,* 2003.

Mikuls TR, Cerhan JR, Criswell LA, Marlino L, Mudano AS, Burma M, Folsom AR, Saag KG. Coffee, tea, and caffeine consumption and risk of rheumatoid arthritis: results from the Iowa women s Health Study. *Arthritis Rheum.* 2002; 46 (1): 83—91.

Miller HE, Rigelhof F, Marquart L, Prakash A, Kanter M. Antioxidant content of whole grain breakfast cereals, fruits and vegetables. *Journal of American Coll. Nutrition* 2000 19(3): 312S—319S.

Manore MM. Finding the Perfect Diet: Revisiting the Pyramid. A Nutritionist View. *ACSM'S Health and Fitness Journal,* 2004; 8(1): 23—26.

Morgan, J. and Morgan, J. *Caribbean Cookbook, Casual and Elegant Recipes*

Inspired by the Islands. Morgan Corporation Limited, 1996.

Morton J. 1987 Black Sapote p. 416—418. in Fruits of warm climates. 2003, At: *www.hort.purdue.edu/newcrop/morton/Black_sapote.html.*

Morton J. 1987 Sapodilla p. 393—398. in Fruits of warm climates. 2003, At: *www.hort.purdue.edu/newcrop/morton/sapodilla.html.*

Muller. HG. *An Introduction to Tropical Food Science.* Cambridge University Press.1988.

Nash, J. Incredible Edibles: an Introduction to wild mushrooms, cherimoya and other remarkable foods. *Essence,* 2002.

National Center for Chronic Disease Prevention and Health Promotion. Defining Overweight and Obesity. 2003, *www.cdc.gov/nccdphp/dnpa/obesity/defining.html.*

National Center for Health Statistics. Prevalence of overweight and obesity among adults: United States, 1999—2000 or at *www.cdc.gov/nchs/products/pubs/hestats/ obese/obse99.html.*

National Institute of Health. Weight cycling NIH Publication No. 95—3901, March 1995.

National Institute of Health. Choosing a safe and successful weight-loss program. NIH Publication No. 94—3700, December 1993.

Norman Van Aken. *The Great Exotic Fruit Book.* Speed Press. 1995.

Novo Nordisk. Healthy eating with diabetes, 2003, *www.novonordisk.co.za/ view.asp?ID=1115.*

Nutrition Action Healthletter: Fantastic Fruit at *www.cspinet.org/nah/fantfruit.html.*

Paganga G, Miller N, Rice-Evans CA. The polyphenolic content of fruit and vegetables and their antioxidant activities. What does a serving constitute? *Free Radical Research* 1999; 30 (2): 153—62.

Pedersen BK, Helge JW, Richter EA, Rohde T, Kiens B. Training and natural immunity: effects of diets rich in fat or carbohydrate. *European Journal of Applied Physiology,* 2000; 82(1—2): 98—102.

Persimmon facts. *www.sofresh.co.nz/persimmon/persimmon_facts.html.*

Pirozzo S, Summerbell C, Cameron C, Glasziou P. Should we recommend low fat diets for obesity? Obesity Review, 2003; 4(2): 83—90.

Ponichtera BJ. *Quick and Healthy Recipes and Ideas.* Volume I, 1991.

Ponichtera BJ. *Quick and Healthy Recipes and Ideas.* Volume II, 1995.

Poppitt SD, McCormick D, Buffenstein R. Short term effects of macronutrients preloads on appetite and energy intake in lean women. *Physiological Behavior* 1998; 64(3): 279—285.

Potter JD, Steinmetz K. Vegetables, fruits and phytoestrogens as preventive agents. *IARC Science Publication* 1996; 139: 61—90.

Raban A, Agerholm-larsen L, Flint A, Holst JJ, Astrup A. Meals with similar energy densities but rich in protein, fat, carbohydrate or alcohol have different effects on energy expenditure, and substrate metabolism but not on appetite and energy intake. *American Journal of Clinical Nutrition* 2003; 77(1), 91—100.

Rahamut, W. *Caribbean Flavors*. Macmillan Publishers, 2002.

Rare Fruit Council, International Inc., *Rare and Exotic Tropical Fruit Recipes*. Miami, Florida 1981.

Rissanen, TH et al. Low Intake of Fruits Berries and vegetables is associated with Excess Mortality in Men: The Kuopio Ischaemic Heart Disease Risk Factor (KIHD) Study. *Journal of Nutrition,* 2003.

Rumpier W, Seals J, Clevidence B, Judd J, Wiley E, Yamamoto S, Komat T, Sawaki T, Ishikura Y, Hosoda K. Oolong tea increases metabolic rate and fat oxidation in men. *Journal of Nutrition* 2001; 131 (11): 2848—52.

Salazar-Martinez, Willet WC, Ascherio A, Manson JE, Leitzmann MF, Stampfer MJ, Hu FB. Coffee consumption and risk for type 2 diabetes mellitus. *Annals of Internal Medicine* 2004; 140 (1): 1—8.

Samaha, F.F., Iqbal N, Sesahdri P, Chican KL, Daily DA, McGrory J, Williams T, Williams M, Gracely E, Stern L. A low carbohydrate as compared with a low fat diet in severe obesity *The New England Journal of Medicine* 2003; 348: 2074—81.

Sanders TA. High versus low fat diets in human diseases. *Current Opinion in Clinical Nutrition and Metabolic Care* 2003; 6(2): 151—155.

Schepers A. Bold new blood pressure guidelines: How diet can help. Environmental Nutrition 2003 July and *www.environmentalnutrition.com*.

Shaw et al. *Tropical and Subtropical Foods*. Agscience, Inc. 1998.

Shields, Donna. *Caribbean Light*. Doubleday.1998

Shields, D. Flavors of the Sun: Caribbean Cuisines. *Restaurants, U.S.A.,* 1997.

Smith J, Goldweber S, Lamberts M, Tyson R, Reynolds JS. Utilization potential for semi-tropical and tropical fruits and vegetables in therapeutic and family diets. Proctor of Florida State Horticultural Society 1983; 96: 241—244.

Soloman, J. Sum, Rum, and Fun. Savoring the Tropical Flavors of Caribbean

Cuisine is the next best thing to being there. *Vegetarian Times,* 1998.

Steinberg FM. Bearden MM. Keen CL. Cocoa and chocolate flavanoids: Implications for cardiovascular health. *Journal of American Dietetic Association* 2003; 103 (2) 215—223.

Stubbs RJ, Van wyk MC, Johnstone AM, Harbron CG. Breakfast high in protein, fat or carbohydrates: effect on within-day appetite and energy balance.

Sun J, Chu YF, Wu X, Liu RH. Antioxidant and antiproliferative activities of common fruits. *Journal of Agricultural Food Chemistry* 2002; 50(25): 7449—54.

The fruit pages: at *www.thefruitpages.com/guavas.shtml,* 2003.

The Glycemic Index *www.shakeoffthesugar.com/pages/576386/index.html,* 2003.

Thorn, B. Passion for Fruit: Chefs Head to the Tropics to feed their desire for the exotic. *Restaurant News,* 2002.

Trager J. *Food Chronology.* Henry Holt and Company 1995.

Trichopoulou, A. et al. Guidelines for the Intake of Vegetables and Fruits: The Mediterranean Approach. *International Journal of Vitamin Nutrition Resources.* 2001.

MacLauchlan. *Tropical Desserts.* Macmillan. 1997.

Tropical Fruit and Vegetable Society of the Redlands, Inc. Homestead, Florida.

Tropical Fruit Growers of South Florida, Homestead, Fl.

Tsi D, Nah AK, Kiso Y, Moritani T, Ono H. Clinical study on the combined effect of capsaicin, green tea extract and essence of chicken on body fat content in human subjects. Journal of Nutrition Science Vitamin logy (Tokyo) 2003; 49 (6): 437—41.

Toussaint-Samat, M. A History of Food. Blackwell Publishers 1994.

Tufts University Health and Nutrition Letter: Bigger Bagels, bigger calories count. Volume 12 number 10: 4.

Tufts University Health and Nutrition Letter: Effect of High-Protein Diets: More Than Just Theory. 2002; 20: 3.

Tufts University Health and Nutrition Letter: Simplifying the advice for slimming down: how to avoid the pitfalls of fad diets. April 1999.

University of Florida, Institute of Food and Agricultural Services (IFAS) Tropical Research and Education Center, Homestead, Florida.

Van Aken, Norman. *The Great Exotic Fruit Book.* Ten Speed Press,1995.

Van t Veer, P. et al. Fruits and Vegetables in the prevention of Cancer and Cardiovascular Disease. *Public Health Nutrition,* 2000.

Vietmeyer, N. Exotic Crops: A Taste of the Future. Readers Digest, 1984.

Volek JS, Westman EC. Very low carbohydrate weight-loss diets revisited. Cleveland Clinic Journal of Medicine. 2002; 69(11): 849—862.

Walsh R. McCarthy J. *Traveling Jamaica with Knife, Fork, and Spoon, A Righteous Guide to Jamaican Cookey.* 1995.

Westerterp-Plantenga Ms, Rolland V, Wilson SA, Westerterp KR. Satiety related to 24 hour diet-induced thermogenisis during high protein/carbohydrate vs. high fat diets measured in a respiratory chamber. *European Journal of Clinical Nutrition* 1999; 53(6): 495—502.

Westerterp-Plantenga MS. The significance of protein in food intake and body weight regulation. *Current Opinion in Clinical Metabolic Care* 2003; 6(6): 635—8.

Wheat Foods Council

¥ USDA Agricultural Research Service. *Journal of the American College of Nutrition,* 2002.

¥ Wyatt H, Grunwald G, Mosca C,. Long term weight loss and breakfast in subjects in the National Weight Control Registry. *Obesity Research* 2002; 10: 78—82.

¥ *Institute of European Food Studies.* Trinity College Dublin 1999.

¥ *Journal of the American Dietetic Association,* 1980.

¥ *University of California at Berkeley Wellness Newsletter.* Jan 2002; USDA, ERS. Food Review, 1999.

¥ *Journal of the American Medical Association,* January 2002

¥ American Kidney Fund, April 25 2002.

¥ *American Heart Association,* Oct 2001.

¥ Centers for Disease Control 2001.

¥ The Asia-Pacific Perspective: Redefining obesity and its treatment. WPRO, WHO, Inl. *Association for the study of Obesity, Int.* Obesity Task Force, 2000.

Whitehead JM, McNeill G, Smith JS. The effect of protein intake on 24—h energy expenditure during energy restriction. *International Journal of Related Metabolic Disorder* 1996; 20 (8): 727—32.

Winter D. There some good in everything, even (Glup!) popular diets. *Environmental Nutrition* 2000; 23(2): 2.

Wisotsky W, Swencionis C. Cognitive approaches in the management of obesity. Adolescence Medicine 2003; 14(1): 37—48.

Wolfe L. *The Cooking of the Caribbean Islands.* Time Life Books, Alexandria VA, 1970.

Woodruff S. *The Good Carb Cookbook, Secrets of Eating Low on the Glycemic Index.* Avery Publishing Group, 2001.

Woodruff S. *Secrets of Cooking for Long Life.* Avery Publishing Group, 1999. *www.tropicalfruitworld.com* Australia, 2003. *www.australiantropicalfoods.com,* 2003.

Yshioka M, St-Pierre S, Drapeau V, Dionne I, Doucet E, Suzuki M, Tremblay A. Effects of red pepper on appetite and energy intake. *British Journal of Nutrition* 1999; 82(2): 115—123.

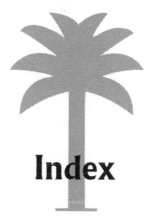

Index

About the Author

Lisa Dorfman, MS, RD, LMHC, registered dietitian, sports nutritionist, and psychotherapist is known nationally as *The Running Nutritionist*™. She has run her own nutrition consulting business, Food Fitness International, Inc. since 1983, and has competed in more than 30 marathons, hundreds of road races, and the Ironman triathlon. She is National Media Spokesperson for The American Dietetic Association.

Lisa is an adjunct professor in the department of exercise science at the University of Miami and is sports nutritionist for the University of Miami Athletic Department's 400+ athletes. Lisa has worked with Olympian athletics, corporate executives, politicians, movie stars, and the infamous housed in the federal correctional system. She has consulted to the cruise and resort industry, launching her Tropical Diet cuisine in the Caribbean over the past few years.

Lisa wrote *The Vegetarian Sports Nutrition Guide* (Wiley, 2000) and has contributed chapters for professional textbooks, sports nutrition guides and feature articles for major magazines. She has been a guest expert for *Dateline, 20/20, CNN, ESPN, MSNBC* and *Fox News* and has appeared in hundreds of publications including *Newsweek, Sports Illustrated for Women, Runners World, Fitness, Muscle & Fitness Hers, Better Homes and Gardens, Glamour, Men's Health, Oxygen, Vegetarian Times,* and *Natural Health.* Lisa is also writing two more books, *The Trauma Diet: A Food, Fitness, and Emotional Recovery Guide* (M. Evans, 2005) and *Anorexia, Bulimia, and Disordered Eating throughout the Lifecycle* (American Dietetic Association, 2005.)

Lisa will be competing in the 2004 World Long Course Duathlon Championships on Team USA in Denmark. Lisa resides in Miami, Florida, with her husband Bob and three children. And, aside from all that, Lisa lives *The Tropical Diet* lifestyle every day.